FLOWER ESSENCES

PLAIN & SIMPLE

LINDA PERRY

THE ONLY BOOK YOU'LL EVER NEED

HAMPTON ROADS

Cover design by Jim Warner
Interior design by Kathryn Sky-Peck

Hampton Roads Publishing Company, Inc.
Charlottesville, VA 22906
Distributed by Red Wheel/Weiser, LLC
www.redwheelweiser.com
Sign up for our newsletter and special offers by going to
www.redwheelweiser.com/newsletter/

*The author and publisher are not responsible for any adverse effects or consequences resulting from
the use of any remedies, procedures, or preparations included herein.
No responsibility is taken for the use of any flower essence, and although all of the essences
mentioned are understood to be safe, they should not take the place of medical treatment
for serious health conditions.*

ISBN: 978-1-57174-765-5

Library of Congress Control Number: 2017934560

Printed in Canada
MAR
10 9 8 7 6 5 4 3 2 1

"Health depends on being in harmony with our souls."

—Dr. Edward Bach

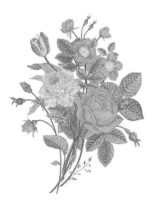

Contents

Part Three:
A Glossary of Essences and Their Uses

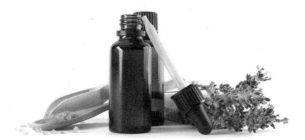

Preface

I am an advanced practitioner and producer of flower and vibrational essences, living in the southwest region of England called Devon, a truly magnificent part of the world where I am surrounded by beautiful and lush English countryside. Devon is very near the county of Cornwall, which is renowned for its magic and mystery. I have lived in this area all my life, as did my ancestors before me, so I have always felt a passionate calling to be aware, to protect, and to learn from the natural world that is around me.

I originally came to work with complimentary therapies as an aromatherapist, but my path developed as I discovered other benefits the natural world had to offer. My work now has expanded to include modalities that are broadly titled vibrational health, specifically the vibrational healing quality of flower essences.

Whereas many holistic therapies target physical health, essences are unique in their ability to work the vibrational or energetic health of an individual, specifically targeting the everyday pressures, stresses, and strains that can leave us not feeling ourselves—mentally, emotionally, and psychically. As a holistic practitioner, I believe in treating the whole individual, which includes the mind, body, and spirit. If these can remain in balance and harmony, then we can truly be healthy and whole. Essences play an important role in the treatment of the whole individual.

All of life around us has a natural way of expressing itself, showing itself, and offering support—everything has an energetic vibration, or life force.

Essences capture these energetic vibrations, so that they can be used as a gentle, practical tool for healing and well-being.

This book will provide you a plain and simple introduction to what flower essences are, how they can be used, and will give you some information on various flowers and plants that you can use for essences. I describe several of the different flower essences I have produced, so you and others may "feel" through my words the difference they can make. When you relate to the plant, its energy, its essence, and understand its message, it will inspire you to begin your own journey on the road to improving your health and well-being. Essences are simply a way to rejuvenate you. They can aid you in working through difficult times, and naturally support and maintain your health in a holistic way.

This book focuses on flower essences, but there are many sources from which an energy signature can be derived and an essence made. Flowers, plants, trees, crystals, colored lasers, colored lights, colored glass, musical instruments, tuning forks, drums, human voices, the sounds of nature—the list is endless! All things have a wavelength and a vibration, which is also a life force. As you grow in your experience working with essences, you will find yourself becoming attuned to the energetic vibrations in things other than flowers and plants.

Bear in mind that the treatment modalities expressed in this book should on no account take the place of medical treatment for a serious health condition, nor should they take the place of professional help and advice if you have any history of mental health challenges.

—Linda Perry

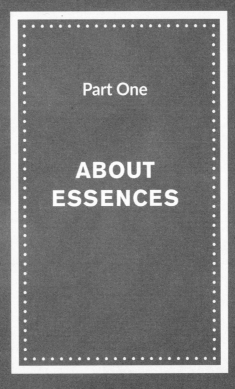

Part One

**ABOUT
ESSENCES**

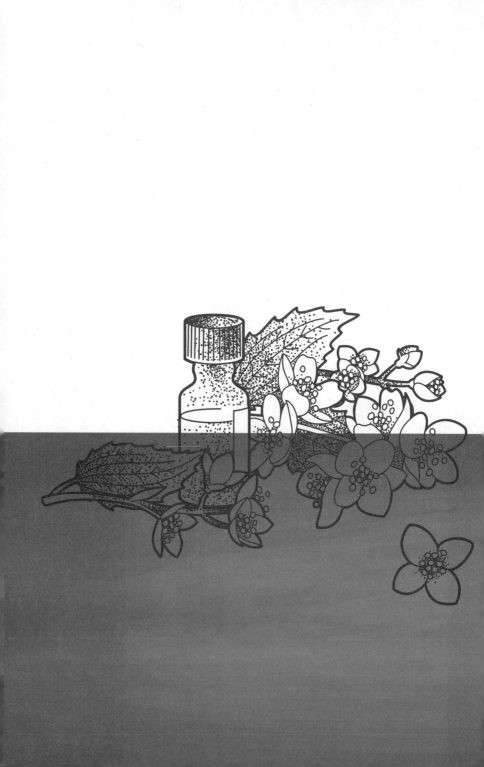

What Are Essences?

1

Most people today are familiar holistic healing therapies, particularly the practice of using herbs for healing. But raise the subject of healing with flower essences, and most people are at a loss to tell you what an "essence" is.

I usually to start by clarifying what essences are *not*. Essences are not the same as essential oils. In fact they are very different. Essential oils are used in aromatherapy treatments, home fragrance, and bath and body products. Unlike essential oils, essences contain no biological material, have no scent, and no confirmed physical therapeutic properties that you would associate with an essential oil used in aromatherapy.

Essences are not homeopathic remedies, nor are they medicinal.

So what are they?

Essences are liquid solutions that contain the energetic or vibrational nature of the flower or plant from which it is made. An essence is the energetic imprint of the life force of the flower or plant. This imprint is captured in water and then a preservative is added (usually alcohol). This solution, or *decoction*, is then stored in bottles (which usually include an eyedropper) so that the essence can be taken orally, added to bath and body products, or used on chakras or meridian points.

Unlike essential oils, essences do not contain any of the biological content of the plant from which they are made; therefore, they are non-toxic.

Essences are simply water and a preservative that holds the energy signature of the particular source (say, a flower). When I am preparing essences, brandy is my preservative preference, but alternatives may be used, such as vodka, vegetable glycerin, or vinegar. The preservative is only used to increase the shelf life of the essence and kill any bacteria that sneak in from opening and closing the bottles.

An Imprint or Energy Signature

It's important to understand what an imprint or energy signature actually is, especially in relation to discussing essences. I believe, as do many others, that nature has its own energy or life force. This energy or life force allows everything around us to function, live, adapt, grow, blend, and flourish within its surroundings, and to survive its environment by evolving to cope with challenges around it.

Many people and cultures refer to this energy or life force by different names. Different cultures may also have varying thoughts and explanations of its working, origins, and meaning. But it may help you to understand the term "life force" by using terms that are more widely shared or known.

Most people are familiar with the word "chi," or "qi," used by the Chinese to describe the life force. The yogis of India refer to the life force as *prana*. The Hawaiians call the life force *mana*. Native Americans call it *manitou*; in Hebrew the life force is known as *ruach*, and in Islamic cultures it is known as *baraka*.

The concept of "life force," by many different names, resonates throughout time, throughout civilizations, countries, and cultures.

All life, in whatever form it takes, comprises energy, and this energy is constantly mixing, merging, and exchanging. People like Isaac Newton and Albert Einstein spent years exploring it through physics and the same goes for those who are studying quantum

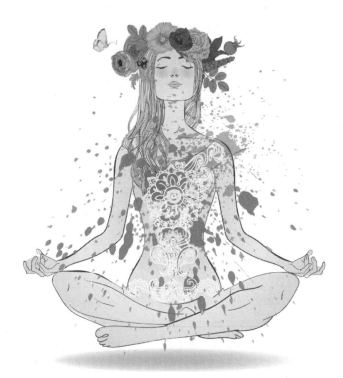

mechanics today—so much in the universe does seem to relate to vibrations and energy. Even popular culture recognizes the concept; how many times have you heard "May the force be with you"?

Essence making is a tool for capturing the vibrations and energies of life. Much research has been done over years by scientists and other people on how water can be affected by vibration and the energy to which it is exposed, and the way that it can hold a memory of the energy or vibrations to which it has been exposed. This is why flower essences are prepared in water.

Subtle Bodies and Subtle Energies

To understand how essences work, you need to recognize that a human being is more than just a physical body. Each person has his or her own external and internal energy and vibrational centers. You may have heard of these described as auras, chakras, subtle bodies, or meridians—to just name a few. Many people simply visualize these energies and vibrations as mists that surround and go through us; they can carry different colors, frequencies, sounds, and speeds. These are not visible to human eye but they are still very much there. Interchanging, mixing, and merging with each other and all living things throughout the world.

Here is a great example of the way in which these subtle bodies and energy centers can impact the way you feel or affect what you think about a situation: Take a moment to think of a time when you met someone and liked them instantly, although you have never met before. How about a time when you have walked into a room and not been comfortable or sure about the space you were in, uncomfortable with the "vibes"? Or a time when you took a walk in nature and experienced a difference in emotion without knowing quite why? This is because your vibration and energy centers mix with the vibrations and energy centers that are around you, affecting your thoughts and feelings, thus creating a vibration and energy within you. Those external and internal energy centers evoke emotional and psychical responses, making you feel a certain way.

Thinking about the body in this way gives you a new, enhanced perspective on health and well-being. Being aware of ourselves as vibrational energy does not take away the fact that we have a physical body, it just extends our notion of ourselves beyond what we can "see."

Our physical and emotional needs will always require our attention, and working with energy and or essences should never be a replacement or alternative to getting medical care and attention. I would like to stress at this point that if you have a condition or illness you should seek out medical help by consulting your own doctor or other health care professional.

Acknowledging that our energy systems can be affected by many things leads us to think of the way that stress, shock, trauma, happiness, or love can affect us. Or how about the physical traumas such as operations, illnesses, and accidents? Add to this such concepts as our diet, surroundings, and environment, as well as electromagnetic items, televisions, computers, and phones. Also just being in nature, around people and animals, can influence how we feel and respond to the world around us.

The lives that we all lead today are fast paced, and sometimes we are forgetful or removed altogether from the natural world, meaning we sometimes we find it difficult to connect or relate to our own life force. We discover that our energy is not as strong as it could or should be. With all the normal everyday things that life throws at us and the emotions we pick up from them, we can sometimes feel unbalanced or not quite our true selves. Imagine or visualize your energy as if it has been knocked or dented, pushed away or even damaged over time due to your feelings or experience of life.

This is where our ancestors had an almost instinctual knowledge of plants and the natural world around them. When our energy systems are affected—whether by thoughts, feelings, or life experience—we can feel off-balance. This is where working with energy and using the life force and the imprint of the vibrations we can obtain through essences can make a difference. We use what nature has to offer, by taking the vibrational energy imprint of the flowers and plant this imprint into our own energy system. The goal is to bring about a natural balance to the vibrations of our mind, body, and soul, so that an optimum state of health and well-being can be achieved. As everything has its own energy, the combination of what to use and when it should be used is unique to each of us.

As a practitioner of vibrational essences, this is what I work with. I am using essences to offer you the energy and vibrations of something special, so that your own energy imprint is improved. This in turn is a way of healing and of taking power over your own general health and well-being.

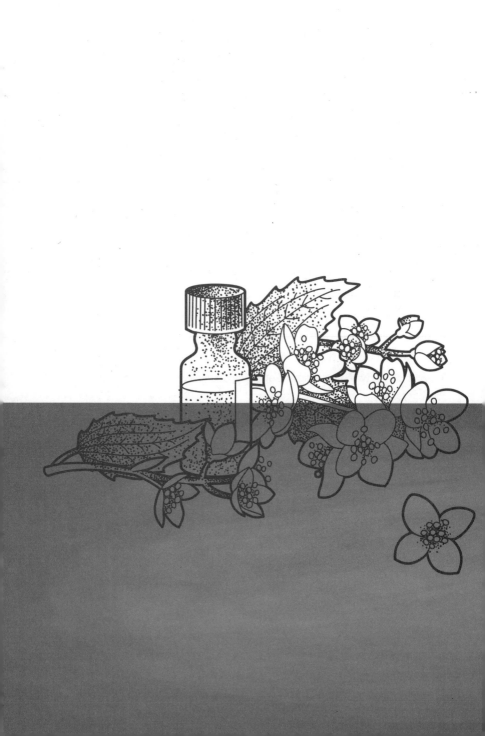

How to
Choose
Essences

2

How do you choose an essence that is right for you? People ask me this all the time, and sometimes the task can appear to be more daunting than the issue they are trying to balance or the things they need help with. Understanding what an essence *is* is one thing. Understanding which to choose is quite another. To help you get started, I have included at the back of this book a glossary of common essences and keywords for the symptoms they treat (see page 103).

But choosing an essence need not be complicated—especially when you take your intellect out of it and learn to trust your intuition. Your body will just "know" what essence it needs for each problem. When you are just starting out working with essences, a statement like this alone is not overly helpful. Remember, however, that when working with essences, you are in the realm of the vibrational energies of life forces—your own vibrations as well as the vibrations of the plants and flowers.

Trusting your own intuition is really the only way forward. It truly is possible to listen and accept that inner voice, to recognize "knowing" without using your rational mind, and without explanation. You need to trust that there may be an unknown vibration swaying you toward essences as a whole, or to one essence in particular.

Here are a few methods that will help you choose an essence for yourself.

Feeling the Energies: Instinct and Intuition

This is my always my first suggestion when choosing essences—trust your intuition. Essences will give a lift to the way you feel, so it makes sense to connect with an essence and check it out to see how it makes you feel. To do this let me give you some suggestions:

- Find a quiet spot where you will not be interrupted or distracted, and ensure you have a pen and paper at hand, as this will help you keep a record of what happens.

- Hold an essence bottle in your hand against your chest, close to your heart, then close your eyes, and take a few deep breaths. Keep breathing deeply for a few minutes, taking the time to rest and relax.

- Now focus on your feet and feel them physically firmly connected to the ground.

- Try to clear your mind of thoughts other than this experience. Stay in this moment of space and time, knowing that all will be as it should.

- When you are ready, ask yourself. how does this essence you are holding actually make you feel?

If you are at a loss, you can help yourself by focusing on the thoughts are bubbling up during this exercise:

- What memories are there for you to access now?

- How does your body feel?

You can also visualize the plant, flower, or source of the essence and see if that brings ideas, inspiration, or guidance:

- For example, visualize a rose. See the color in your mind, conjure up a memory of the smell of the rose.

- What immediately comes to mind? Love? Peacefulness? Perhaps pain or rejection?

In all of these exercises, write down some keywords for each essence that you can refer to later.

It's important to avoid over analyzing things at this time; instead, try to focus on the essence alone, and allow the life force within the bottle to connect itself to you. If you start to doubt what you are feeling, put the bottle down, push it away from you, and try another bottle.

By allowing yourself to tune in to such subtle factors, and by trusting your inner voice, you will soon learn to recognize the essences that resonate with your own energy systems. Amazingly, you will soon know if this essence will help you feel the way you want to.

Although intuition and instinct are your most valuable tools, knowledge and intellect can also help in choosing an essence. If you happen to be in a space and time where clear thoughts and comprehension of your feelings are not possible, or you are finding it difficult to access or experience your feelings, you can simply read the manufacturer's description of the essence and see if the words mean something to you. If they do, the message will be clear.

Dowsing with a Pendulum

Because essences have an energy signature or vibration, another way you can check if an essence is right for you is to visually measure it against your own energy. A very simple way to do this is to dowse. As a practitioner, this is one of my favorite ways to work with people, because it allows you to feel and see your own energies.

In order to dowse you will need some sort of pendulum. A pendulum is simply a weight suspended from a chain or string, and which is allowed to swing freely. Your pendulum could be a special purchase—there are many different varieties available—or it could be a pendulum you make from a favorite necklace, or simply a homemade arrangement that you make by tying the end of a piece of string around a stone or crystal.

How does it work? Think of the pendulum as a tool that picks up information from the unseen vibrations around and within us. The pendulum connects with the vibrations and energy waves emitted from either our thoughts, those of other people, and from places, crystals, foods, flowers, animals, and much more. These energies can't be seen, but the pendulum creates a bridge between the logical and intuitive parts of the mind, and it allows us to see the effects of the life force within whatever we are testing and it can give us visual confirmation when needed.

A common misconception is that dowsing will only work if you are psychic or unusually sensitive to unseen forces. This simply isn't true; there is nothing magical or mystical about dowsing. We are simply using the pendulum to allow us to see the vibration for ourselves. Weird as this may be, so many people are amazed at the accuracy of dowsing that they often see the process as some kind of magic.

How to Dowse

Start by making yourself comfortable. Then hold your pendulum in one hand by the chain or string and hold it still. Keep your hand and arm relaxed, because tensing up will prevent the pendulum from swinging freely.

Take a moment to ask a question in your mind or speak it out loud—the option is yours. Make sure the question you ask can be answered by a simple "yes" or "no." For example, I would ask, "Is my name Linda?" I know the answer to this is yes, so then I would watch the pendulum to see how it responds.

There is usually some movement that you can see, but you may need to practice for a while at first, so give yourself time and don't worry about the outcome. Note the way the pendulum moves; for instance, for me the pendulum will give a "yes" answer by swinging in a clockwise circle. For others it will move in the other direction or up and down or from side to side. There is no right or wrong because the results are unique to each person.

Now try a question where the answer is a definite "no." I usually ask, "Is my name Mickey Mouse?" and watch the movement change. It will move in a different way. For me it will now go counter-clockwise. Once you have established your "yes" and "no" movements of response you can start to ask other questions.

Remember we are checking the answers with our bodily vibrations, and we are not expecting the pendulum to be moved by a supernatural force. It is simply a matter of it responding to small unconscious muscle movements in your arm (this is a form of kinesiology). Through this method, you are accessing your own truth without needing to use your logical mind. The pendulum is providing a bridge, a way of allowing you to access your own internal knowledge and intuition.

Take some time to really think about what you want from your essence, and consider what you would like it to do. Try and set an *intention* so that next time you work with an essence, you will know what you are asking for and where you most need clarification or something to lean on. If this has succeeded, you are ready to work with an essence.

Dowsing for Essences

You can hold the essence bottle in one hand and hold the pendulum in the other hand so that it is directly over the essence. Ask yourself, "Is this essence right for me?" The "yes" or "no" answer given by your pendulum will be your answer.

It helps to set your intention on the outcome that you want from the essence. I say this because many essences can be "right," but not necessarily right for the stage of life that you are at currently. So before starting, ensure you take a moment to think about what you want to know *now*. Then you can ask, "Is this essence right for me?" You will get a more accurate answer this way.

Muscle Testing

Another way of selecting your essence, and determining what your body/mind needs, is through muscle testing. You can do this in many ways, but my preference for self-testing is to use the fingers. A practitioner can do this for you, but the method I describe below can be done *by* you *for* you.

- Start by making yourself comfortable.

- Press your thumb and forefinger together to make a circle.

- Now use the forefinger of the opposite hand and try and break the circle.

Obviously unless you are fighting against yourself, you are always going to be able to break the circle. Try not to think about the action of actually breaking the circle but more the recognition of the force it took to do it. As with the dowsing, think of something that is true, and test a result. Then do the same with a lie. If the circle breaks easily the answer is "no" and if it gives a little resistance the answer is "yes."

To put this muscle technique to use, bring a bottle of essence into your energy circle, within your aura. You can do this by putting on the table in front of you, or by holding it in your hand. Now with a clear intention of your situation and of the outcome you are trying to achieve, ask the same question: "Is this essence right for me?"

As before, you are looking for subtle differences that your own true feelings and intuitions are telling you through the experiences of small muscle movements, strength, and resistance.

There are many other methods people use and no one method, in my opinion, is right or wrong. You are the best judge of what you feel you can use and what outcome you can trust. So my advice is to choose the method that suits you and feels right for you. Of course, you can contact a registered essence practitioner or professional for further advice and help.

If you are really sensitive to energies, you can even hold your hand over each bottle and see what you get from it—your hand may start to tingle, or feel warm.

Or you could enlist the help of a friend when trying muscle testing. Hold the essence in your hand and stretch your arm out to one side. Then ask your friend to push your arm down. It if goes down easily, the essence is not right for you; if the arm stays put despite your friend's efforts, it is right for you.

Using the above methods, you may find that more than one essence connects with your needs. In the following chapters we will discuss how to make essences, and what the benefits of each essence may be.

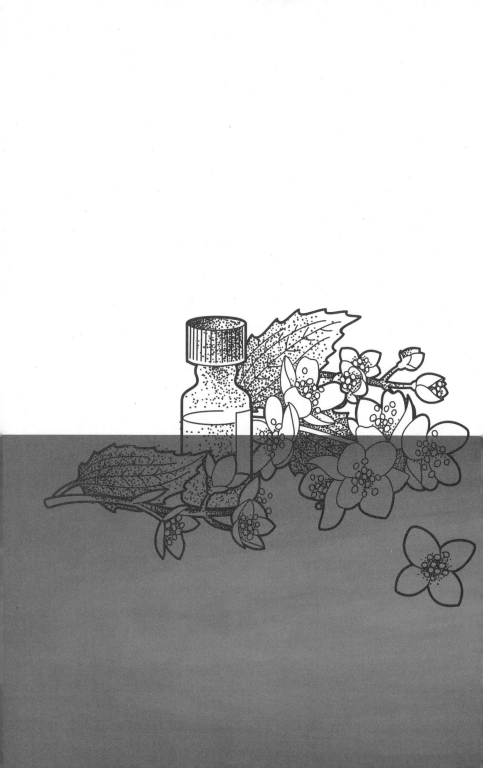

How to Make a Bottle of Essence

3

You may wonder if essences come in different strengths, but the answer is no. Essences are an energy signature or a life force, so they aren't something that can be measured. You may however hear terms such as mother essence, stock essence, and dosage essence.

I am going to explain the difference so that you can understand how to make up bottles of essence, or indeed how bottles that you buy may have been made up.

Mother Essence

A *mother essence* is the first source of actual essence made by the producer, and consists of the water used in the making the essence and a preservative. A mother essence is not used directly. Mother essences can be made in a variety of different ways.

The most widely known and accepted method is the sunlight method. In this method, a bowl of water is placed in direct sunlight with the source of the essence—for example flower blooms—placed gently into the water. This open bowl is left in the sunlight for a period of time, and then is decanted, filtered, and stored in a preservative of choice—usually brandy—at a one to one ratio of water to preservative. The period of time the bloom is left in the sunlight varies from one producer to the next, but generally the length of time is three hours.

Many people prefer an alcohol-free essence. You can substitute an equal amount of vegetable glycerin (found online) or apple cider vinegar in place of the brandy.

There are also some essences that are made in moonlight. This is exactly like the sunlight method, but the bowl of water is instead placed in the moonlight.

There are many adaptations to these two basic methods. Sometimes a crystal is placed in the water and essence is drawn from that. Some essences are made from the morning dew that comes from the plants, rather than the plant itself. Some essences are made in sunlight and have moon-energized water added later. There are a wide variety of methods to explore, and the method will come to you intuitively, and through practice.

Stock Essence

From the mother essence comes the *stock essence.* This is an essence made in a new bottle filled with water and preservative, to which some of the mother essence is added. The actual amount of mother essence added will vary from producer to producer, but to give you an idea of the ratio, it is often two to seven drops of mother essence per 20 to 30 ml bottle. Stock essences are usually the type of bottled essences that you can purchase from shops or online. A stock essence can be taken directly under the tongue or a few drops can be added to a glass of water; each producer will have his or her own suggestion on the number of drops to add. This information will be detailed on the label.

Dosage Essence

Dosage essences are kept separate and are different from the mother and stock. Dosage bottles are usually filled with approximately 50 percent water and 50 percent preservative, with only a few drops of the stock essence added, so it is more dilute than the stock essence. This allows an individual to take the essence under the tongue or added to water, and it is generally assumed that this is a more palatable way to ingest an essence, or possibly a kinder and gentler way of using essences because you can absorb the essence at intervals throughout the day as needed. It is also a matter of economy, since it is a way of making essences last longer.

The main benefit, however, of a dosage essence is that it allows you to take a variety of essences together in a combination. When you are selecting an essence for a particular situation or intention, you may find that more than one essence is indicated for you. In this case, you would require a combination dose, and the more diluted essences are perfect for these combinations.

The Indirect Method

When a plant is poisonous—and many plants are—the only way to prepare an essence from it is by the *indirect method*. Unlike the direct method, in which the source flower is actually put into the water, the indirect method captures the energy signature by its proximity to the water. The plant or flower is placed next to the bowl of water as it sits in the sunlight or moonlight.

This is sometimes also called the *environmental method*. In some cases, the plant isn't poisonous but the person making the essence prefers to leave the plant to grow where it is. This is a good way to make use of rare or wild plants.

In the indirect method, a bowl of water is placed in a particular location or within proximity of the source of energy, such as a sacred site or a natural wonder such a waterfall or remote natural beauty spot. The water could be placed near huge tidal waves or by calming seas, or yet again, in extreme climates such as rain-forest or mountains. The list is endless, because in this case, the energy of the environment is being captured in the water.

Other Considerations

Oftentimes other considerations are taken in account when making essences. Essences can add special attributes depending on when they are made, such as being made on a specific date, during a certain moon alignment, during a certain season, or a particular time of day. If you are pagan or an astrologer, you may give special consideration to the moon phase, or the astrological sign or aspect. This is a personal choice for the person producing or taking the essence, and may enhance the experience of making and using essences.

No Contraindications

Flower and vibrational essences have no known contraindications since there is no raw (biological) material found in the mother essence or any subsequent stock or dosage essences. So, for instance, if you are allergic to almonds you can still take almond essence if needed. The essences can be used for the elderly, for children, and animals, as well as in combination with other medications you may be taking (but please discuss this with your health practitioner first).

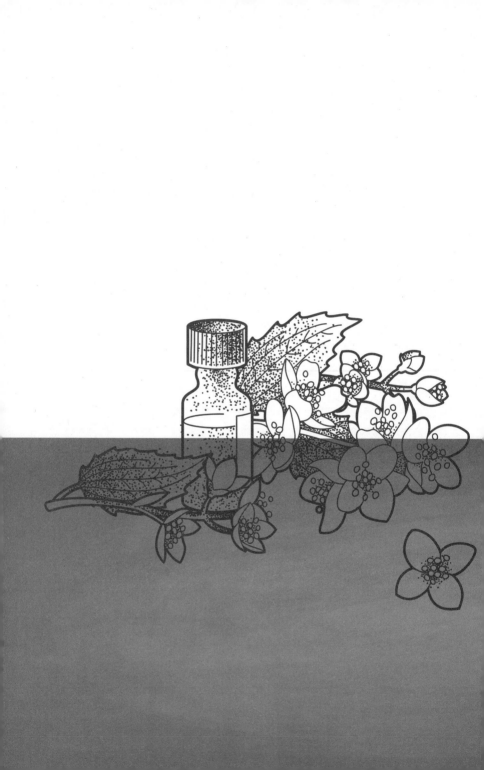

Essences, Chakras, and Subtle Bodies

4

We have talked about the fact that essences capture the vibrational energy signature of the plant or flower from which they are made, but they are used to affect your *own* vibrational energy signature or life force. This chapter will review some of the concepts you need to know to understand your own life force.

The Chakras

Chakras are internal energy centers that cannot be seen with our eyes. There are several cultural belief systems as to exactly how they work and how they respond, and there are a variety of names and attachments given to them. A common belief is that each chakra is a capsule of energy, holding, vibrating, outputting, and maintaining our energy and unique life force. When the chakras are vibrating in balance with each other, we feel at our best. Following are the seven main chakras, and the basic properties of each of them.

Root Chakra

The Root Chakra is found at the base of the spine, and it is often associated with the color red. It is the area connected to our place on earth, and to what keeps us grounded and secure. So the emotions and energies attached to things such as family, finances, home life, relationships, and survival vibrate here.

Sacral Chakra

The Sacral Chakra is found just below the naval, and is often associated with the color orange. It is the area connected to the

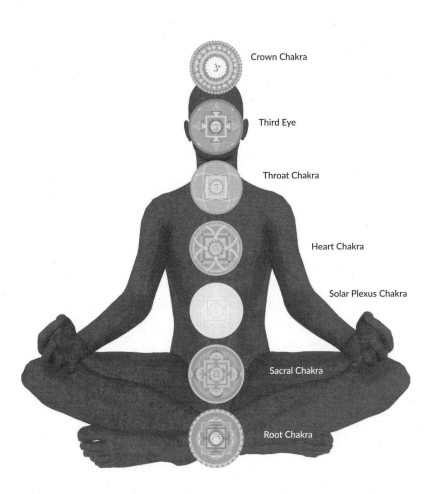

Crown Chakra

Third Eye

Throat Chakra

Heart Chakra

Solar Plexus Chakra

Sacral Chakra

Root Chakra

emotions, our gut instincts, and subtle senses that are attached to your sexuality, creativity, and passion.

The Solar Plexus Chakra

The Solar Plexus Chakra is found just above the navel, and this area is associated with the color yellow. It is the area that connects to our will power, empowerment, and control. Emotions such as fear are influenced here.

The Heart Chakra

The Heart Chakra is found close to the heart area and it is associated with the colors pink or green. It is the area that connects to desire, love, and compassion. It is also linked to emotions such as loneliness.

The Throat Chakra

The Throat chakra is found in the throat area and is associated with the color blue. It is the area connected to expression, communication, and trust, and so connected to such things as saying what we consider to be the truth, but also with confidence or the lack of it, and doubt.

The Third Eye

The Third Eye Chakra is found in the center of the forehead, and the color associated to this area is indigo. It is an area attached to knowledge, insight, intuition, and faith, and as such linked to clarity, focus, and perception.

The Crown Chakra

The Crown Chakra is found just above the head and it is associated with the color violet. This is the area that attaches to the soul's purpose, spiritual connection, and divine purpose, thus to inspiration, intuition, and a sense of completeness.

The Subtle Bodies

Some consider that there are as many subtle bodies as there are chakras. Working outward from our physical bodies, we are surrounded by copies of the physical body, but in an energy form. These energy shapes are called subtle bodies, and while they are always slightly away from our physical body, they hold the vibration that is carried within and around us. Like our chakras they are vibrating, outputting, and maintaining our energy and our unique life force, and when we regain balance in these bodies, we find our holistic health and well-being improve.

The subtle bodies that I work with and refer to can be seen as auras of mist around the body, and working outward from the physical form, they vary in size, shape, and speed of movement. If you want to give them names, you can visualize them as the following:

The Etheric Subtle Body

The etheric subtle body is almost a blueprint copy of the physical form and it is the energy center that is most likely to be first affected by any shock or trauma. It supports and holds our feelings, and under normal circumstances allows us to feel secure. Like the base chakra, it concerned with fears, insecurities, and sensations of loss or disorganization, indecision, and the need to be grounded and functioning.

The Emotional Subtle Body

Then we have the emotional subtle body, which is linked to energies that harken back to unresolved issues, severe emotional trauma, and relationships that may be good or bad. This also links to acceptance, change, anger, frustration, and happiness.

The Mental Subtle Body

Then we have mental subtle body, which is linked to our thoughts, ideas, knowledge, and wisdom. It is where we hold feelings associated to self-definition, will, positivity, boundaries, beliefs, ego, and self-worth.

The Causal Subtle Body

The causal subtle body is related to communication, self-expression, inspiration, guidance, confidence, suppressed emotions and personal destiny.

The Soul Subtle Body

Next is the soul subtle body, which is coupled with attachment, habit, and approach to life, along with faith, purpose, and intuition.

The Spiritual Subtle Body

Lastly the spiritual subtle body is attached to our awareness, our ability to feel, and live our life purpose.

Understanding the vibrations of plants and flowers and understanding your own vibration energy are the two pieces of the puzzle to using essences. Essences can make a real difference to your emotional, mental, spiritual health, and well-being. I would like to encourage you to understand and give the reasons why a certain plant, flower, crystal or other source may have been chosen, and then the manner in which it may influence your own energy centers and life force.

There are hundreds of essences available, more than the scope of this book can cover. But this is a plain and simple introduction to flower essences, and in the next section, you find information on essences that have been made from flowers, trees, and plants. I have had experience making all of these essences myself, and I have chosen these particular essences because it's easy for me to discuss their message and to tell you their story.

Note: I mentioned it before but I make no apology for mentioning it again. Using essences is by no means an alternative for seeking medical care or attention. Please consult your doctor if you are at all worried about your health. You might wish to ask your doctor his or her thoughts and experiences with essences, as many doctors and pharmacists do have experience of using them and prescribing them.

Getting to know a plant and connecting with it in this way will give you invaluable insight on what the plants message might be. So let's step into the world of essences and find out more.

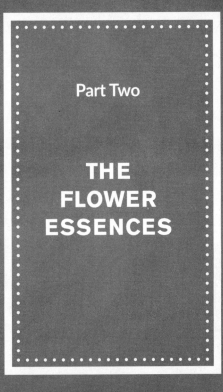

Part Two

THE
FLOWER
ESSENCES

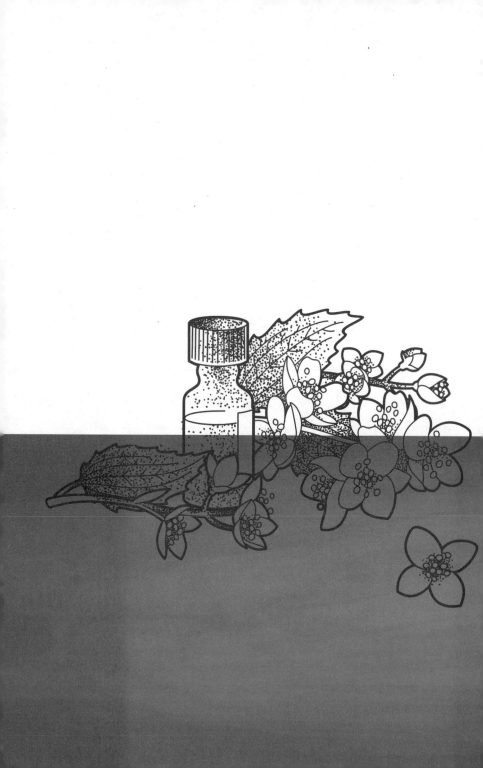

Essence Pioneer
Dr. Edward
Bach

5

It is impossible to discuss flower essences without introducing this remarkable gentleman. Dr. Edward Bach was a British physician, pathologist, bacteriologist, homeopath, writer, and founder of the Bach Flower Remedies. He was born on September 24, 1886, and he studied and practiced orthodox medicine for many years. He had a very successful clinic in the famous doctor's street in London, Harley Street, but soon found himself challenging the fact he was just treating the physical disease or symptom and not the whole person. He believed that a patient's state of mind and emotions should also be considered; he observed that when someone was struggling emotionally, this would have a damaging impact on the physical self as well.

Dr. Bach started researching a natural and supportive way of bringing help, which led him to research and document many different negative states of mind. He specifically defined seven moods that cause disease and suffering: fear, uncertainty, loneliness, lack of interest, over-sensitivity, over-concern for others, and despair. He then went on to discover a total of thirty-eight different flowers that could help bring about changes for his patients. He defined the seven qualities of healing disease as hope, peace, faith, joy, certainty, love, and wisdom.

He spent the spring and summer months making essences, while treating people in the winter months often free of charge. He truly believed the mind played an important part in improving general health and well-being, and he wanted to make this his life's work and inspire others to look at their health in this way. He wanted to bring a spiritual sense of purpose and a joy back to people's lives and he helped many people in this way up to his death in 1936.

Dr. Bach's writings and treatments have been well documented and shared, and I encourage you to research the work he has done, and read any one of his many books so that you may embrace the legacy that he left behind. We can remind ourselves that nature is there to help. It won't change who we are but it can relieve and support us through life's events.

Dr. Bach's work certainly inspired me as I worked to research and use the flower essences in the following chapters. So with this in mind, I share with you some of Dr. Bach's own words, hoping they will inspire you to research and explore your own interest in essences.

"The action of these remedies is to raise our vibrations and open up our channels for the reception of our Spiritual Self, to flood our natures with the particular virtue we need, and wash out from us the fault which is causing harm. They are able, like beautiful music, or any gloriously uplifting thing which gives us inspiration, to raise our very natures, and bring us nearer to our Souls: and by that very act bring us peace and relieve our sufferings. They cure, not by attacking disease, but by flooding our bodies with the beautiful vibrations of our Higher Nature, in the presence of which disease melts as snow in the sunshine."

—Collected Writings of Edward Bach (1987, p. 117)

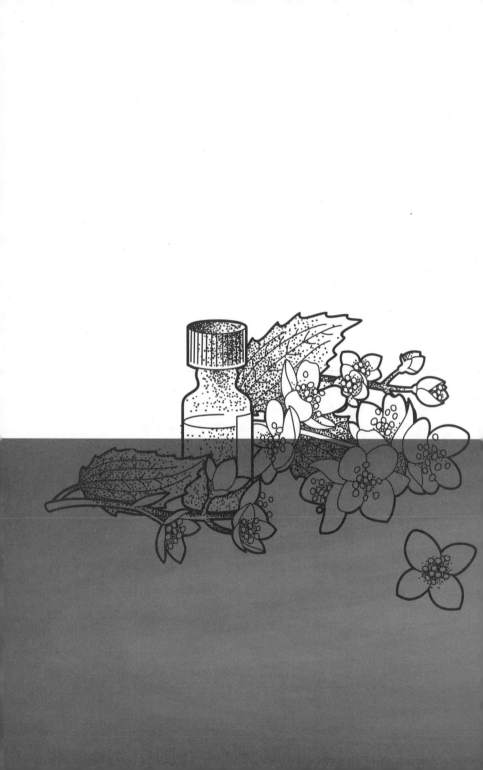

Cream Rose
Essence

6

*"I allow all to be in balance, to
feel surrounded above, below, and
beyond in a bubble of love."*

Spend some time with a rose and get to know its characteristics and traits, as this will give you clues to what the essence may bring. Just take a moment to think of a rose, or consider finding a real plant, and sit with and look at one that you can touch, feel, and smell. Alternatively, you can study a picture in detail or perhaps an essence that has already been made. There are many different kinds of rose, and as such I think they have many messages to share.

Let us start let by looking at the way in which they grow. A rose is a perennial, so it will grow, flower, and seed through one season and then carry on doing so for future years. This gives you a unique insight to its life force, which in this example, denotes the rose's ability to recreate and renew itself. A rose could be a climber, a bush, or a tree, and it might be wild or specially cultivated. How it grows will give you an insight to the way that the energy signature is directed in the plant. For example if it is a low, sturdy, grounded shrub, it is bound to have an energy signature that talks of being very grounded and sturdy. On the other hand, it may be a tall and rampant climber, constantly striving higher, bringing an energy signature of a goal setter or high achiever. It may have varied branches of varied lengths, all covered with prickles and thorns, suggesting a need for protection.

When cream rose presented herself to me, I found her to have long branches and huge cream flower blooms. Most roses have a wonderful scent that they use to attract insects to their pollen, but also to attract people and animals for pleasure, interest, and enjoyment. This was certainly the case for me, and it tells the story of how I spotted this particular cream rose. She had an amazingly sweet scent, like vanilla ice-cream, and huge blooms as

Cream rose

that were big as my hand. As far as I know she was not purposely planted but growing wild.

Roses are found in many colors, and because colors have many connections to the way in which we see and feel the world, color becomes important. For example, had my rose been red, it might have represented passion and love, or if it had been orange, maybe a zest of life and enthusiasm. Yellow could have suggested creativity and friendship, white might have indicated purity and peace, or pink denoting appreciation or confidence. However, this rose was cream, so it felt feminine, delicate, warm, caring; yet strong and determined to be spotted.

Looking closer at shape of these blooms in detail showed me they were many circular domes that were flamboyant and frilly. The domes held many droplets of water until too full, then each dome acted as a small cup, allowing the water to cascade gently down one section, one petal and one stage at a time, until ready for release. While this could be interpreted in many ways, the message I took from it was the ability to both hold and release, to hide and be open, to change and transform. This would most certainly come forward in this rose's essence.

The size and quantity of the cream rose blooms was large, but size, of course, can vary depending on the species. A rose bloom can be from one to five inches in diameter or more, and one stem can have one bloom or many. This variation suggests this energy signature could represent individualism and confidence or community and support.

The structure of the branches and the main stem of a rose may be thick or thin, but most are strong and sturdy, holding the weight of one or many blooms. This gives the impression that the blooms seem defy gravity; my impression is that from deep within the plant comes strength, the ability to overcome difficulties, the ability to produce, flourish, evolve, and stand out. The message that comes out of this essence is that it brings power back to your core and to your emotional heart center, and it allows you to feel that inner empowerment.

If I turn my attention to the leaves of the plant, I see that they are ovate and different shades of green. This gives me the message of simplicity, without division, and total balance. The variety of green suggests renewal and regrowth, healing and health.

Roses have long been associated with love, joy, celebration, and beauty. We find mention of them in modern texts but also in ancient texts from Greek, Roman, and Egyptian mythology. Roses are used to express emotion, the flourish in all forms of art, and they have been used in this way for a very long time.

My thoughts and feedback for this essence, and all I have come to know about the rose family, was that it represented energetic recovery and renewal. Everyone needs help when faced with life's transitions, and the essence of this cream rose seems perfect for those unexpected events—especially those that heighten our emotional state, such as shock, trauma, grief, loss, separation, anger, fear, surprise, stress, tension, and the sense of being overwhelmed.

The cream rose brings about a sense of balance, love, and purity. It relaxes and calms us. It helps us think clearly, comforts us, and restores our equilibrium. It can also give a sense of protection, care, health, confidence, serenity, hope, and positivity.

Cream rose is, therefore, my essence of choice for recovery and renewal. I have found it a great all round essence for those who find themselves in situations where they can't focus clearly. Sometimes people can't really work out what is going on inside themselves or perhaps they just feel incomplete.

This essence can be used when you want to tend to your inner sweetness and be admired for who you are without making a spectacle of yourself or attracting undue attention. This is an essence for when you need to be reminded of who you are and how you shine, and of your own unique presence into the world. It allows you to remain strong and supported, cared for and rested, with the opportunity of new beginnings.

The life force of this plant can be felt. It is easy to understand and share in its energy either by being in its presence or through its essence. Either way, you are feeling its vibration.

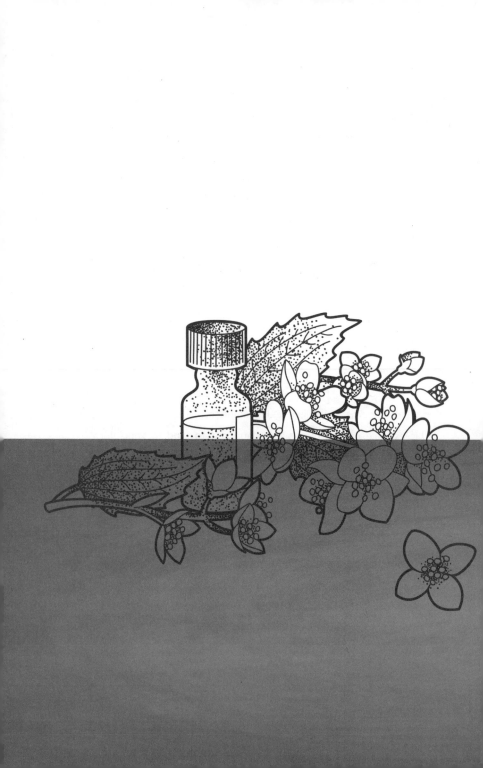

Red Geranium
Essence

7

"I am resilient, stable, protected,
and encouraged."

When you meet a geranium you cannot help but feel how robust these plants actually are. Their stems are chunky little trunks, almost tree-like in strength, from which sprout the leaves, usually in an abundance of evergreen masses. Strong and thriving are qualities I feel are brought to the essence. Every stage of the plant from the roots upward strives forward into the world as it reaches up and out, wanting to be safe but also seen.

This essence injects a sense of strength into your energy fields and fuels your energy and emotional centers, heightening the emotions that are attached to drive, stamina, passion, and vitality. The plant itself demonstrates this: although there are many varieties of geranium, this particular one is an evergreen perennial, meaning that it should last more than two years and flowers annually. I actually bought a geranium plant at a local flower market many years ago and it is still going strong, which is a testament to its endurance.

The bright red color of this plant is connected, via the root chakra, to our core principles and our place in the world. It relates to the way we feel about things like our family, our home, our finances, and the security we receive in life, not only due to our physical necessities being met, but through our relationships. It is connected to a sense of safety and our emotional foundations, all of which are linked to our root chakra and the emotions that we hold here. The red color adds to the vibrational energy to these areas, and it is actually why I chose to use this variety of plant instead of the other color varieties of geranium.

Red geranium essence is about resilience, and the force that propels us forward through life's challenges as we work toward our goals or intentions. It allows us to feel firm in our decisions, to

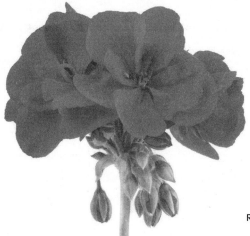

Red geranium

know the way forward, and to overcome challenges of the mind. When we have a firm base, we can stride out into the world just like the zestful geranium plant itself does.

This life force makes geranium the perfect essence if you are finding it hard to get going, or if you need or want to stand out. The geranium plant has long stems that hold a mass of flowers well above the foliage that lies below, and the flowers are made up lots of little tiny spheres that are just wanting to be seen. They will flower until the first frost, so here in the United States and Great Britain, geraniums have a long flowering period—and that is longer still in the milder regions of the country. Throughout its growing period, it can flower many times and regrow where necessary while being nurtured and sustained by the base below. When it has finished its work for the season, it recharges itself from the earth and comes back with the same strength the following year. This essence brings forth a sense of striving enthusiastically toward any goal. The red color drives us forward and the textured robust petals bring forth the energy of determination and passion for success.

It can also be a very protective essence to our subtle bodies, so if you are working with groups of people or if you are very empathetic to your surroundings, it can create a sense of security. The red color brings an emotional warning about overwhelming energies that do not serve us and it prevents stress or anger from sparking into life by balancing our internal vigor. Red geranium allows passion, joy, and love to come to the forefront.

If you are emotionally lethargic, inactive, or lacking motivation, this essence can help. All of its qualities combine to give an energetic kick-start and to lead the way. It encourages us to find the confidence to release the leader within ourselves, so we can become the masters of our own destiny and to feel fully supported by whatever surrounds us.

Remember that when you work with essences, you are using them as a tool that allows the essence of that plant to influence your mood. So why not take a moment to connect with the plant, and see how it makes you feel. Connecting with the actual plant will give you the best results, but if you can't find a plant, a picture of a geranium may give you some insight as to whether this essence is right for you. Try searching for geraniums on the Internet, and you'll find lots of pictures to look at.

Once you have your plant or picture, find a quiet space where you will not be disturbed and ensure that any technology such as phones are turned off.

Close your eyes, take five deep breaths in and out, clearing your mind. Feel your feet on the floor and make a little note to yourself as to the way your physical body feels. Pass no judgment on it—just acknowledge the sensations.

Make note of your emotional state, but don't over-analyze this—just give yourself a score from one to ten, and acknowledge your feelings without judging yourself.

Now move your awareness to your breathing again. Take five breaths in and out again, and slowly open your eyes and look at the plant. How does the plant look? Really look at it in detail, take your time to watch and examine it, and see if you are able to observe all that it is for about ten minutes. Consider its smell, color, shape, height, width, movements, and location.

Then close your eyes again, and take five deep breaths in and out.

How has the plant made you feel? Do any words come to mind right away? Once you have considered this, take five deep breaths in and out, and make a little note to yourself of the way that your physical body feels now.

How do you feel emotionally? Give yourself a score from one to ten.

Consider whether anything has changed as a result of connecting briefly with the plant. You will be able to take any message that has come, so the trick is to trust your inner wisdom and your own counsel and understand what message the geranium has given you.

I like to record my experiences so that I can reflect on them later, so I write them down after the event. Sometimes the messages don't come right away, but reveal themselves to our consciousness later in time.

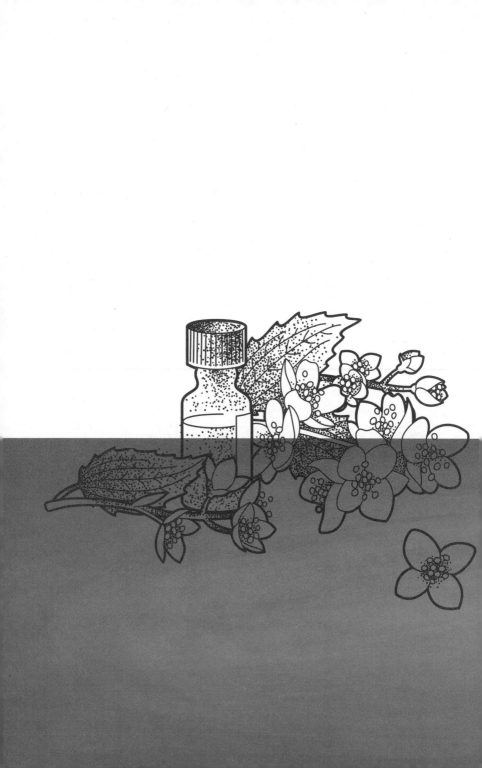

Eucalyptus
Essence

8

*"I am perfectly balanced and
flowing through my life with
grace and ease."*

This essence was the first tree essence that I was drawn to make. I bought the tree as a sapling, nurturing it in a half barrel for around eight years before it became too big for the pot, and then I planted it in the ground. This tree is mesmerizing to watch but when I do, it gives me a clear message of its essence.

A eucalyptus tree is really strong and flexible, and it can bend over with grace and ease without snapping. Mine is in a fairly windy location and sometimes bends over from one side to the other, and sometimes gives the impression of being made of rubber. It look as though it will break and fall over but it doesn't. Eucalyptus grows very quickly, and it is very adaptable to its surroundings. It's a hardy tree that can survive everything from drought, forest fires, hungry animals, and bugs, and when it does become damaged, it grows back quickly

Eucalyptus essence brings emotional cleansing, regrowth, and encouragement when we need a fresh start. Just as the tree behaves in the wind, the essence aids us when we need to bend and change, to be flexible and to go with the flow with complete grace, acceptance, and peace.

This essence inspires us to be strong but not rigid and to continue to grow, develop, and succeed. Therefore, this essence is perfect for times when you feel overwhelmed by emotions, under pressure, or stressed, and you long to clear the clutter out of your head, or you desperately need a fresh start.

The bark of the tree is often light brown or even faintly rainbow colored, and most eucalyptus usually shed their bark at least once a year. The one that I grow certainly does. The impression that I get from this essence is of the tree's cycle of growth and regrowth, so it seems to bring a transformational energy to the

Eucalyptus

essence. Thus eucalyptus clears old patterns and outworn habits, and it allows memories to be stored without attachment to emotions that no longer serve a purpose. The essence is about being in the *present*. It is about clear thinking, cleansing, and refreshing the energies.

The tree has lance-like leaves that are long, thin, and pointed. The menthol in the leaves gives them a bluish tint, which can actually give a forest of eucalyptus a blueish appearance at certain times of the year, as in the great forest of eucalyptus that cover the Blue Mountains to the west of Sydney in Australia.

Green is associated with the heart chakra and blue with the throat chakra, so eucalyptus essence becomes a symbol of our emotions and the way in which we communicate with others. It allows us to release and let go of attitudes that no longer support our dreams and desires. This essence helps with blockages in relationships, expressing oneself, self-confidence, and individual trust that comes from within. All this is connected with our throat chakra, so if we find this area out of balance, we may experience reactions such as anger, anxiety, frustration, fear, irritability, or a build-up of resentment. This essence can strengthen and balance the throat chakra to bring positive qualities to how we release and express our thoughts and feelings with others.

As one of earth's most ancient trees, eucalyptus seems to bring forth an impression of gentle wisdom and knowledge, which allows us to feel cohesive and safe within our own subtle bodies.

Take some time to learn how to connect with your own subtle bodies; the following exercise is a good one for becoming more sensitive to them. Do this exercise in bare feet in a safe spot, preferably outdoors. Doing the exercise indoors will still work, although not perhaps quite as quickly or easily.

Take a moment to stand still and feel your physical body, feel your feet on the ground and use the following verbal meditation:

I feel my toes on the ground

I feel my feet on the ground

I feel my ankles

I feel my legs

I feel my knees

I feel my thighs

I feel my hips

I feel my abdomen

I feel my chest

I feel my shoulders

I feel my arms

I feel my wrists

I feel my fingers

I feel my neck

I feel my throat

I feel my face

I feel my ears

I feel my eyes

I feel my head

While doing this, take your time and breathe in and out between each step of the way.

Now close your eyes and feel those parts of your body that float just a couple inches away from your physical body. Visualize them as white mists surrounding you. Run through the meditation elements again, but see them in your mind's eye a couple inches away from your body. Remember to breathe and take your time. Now run through it again, going out a few additional inches away from your body. Repeat this exercise, gradually moving further out each time, until you feel that you are at the extreme edge of your comfort zone. In my experience, the more we practice this exercise, the further way we can feel and understand our subtle bodies.

Soon afterward, when you come into contact with things that influence those subtle bodies, you will recognize them and acknowledge them, and this will help keep everything in balance. This will also help when you wish to use an essence that you have already chosen or when you want to find one for a specific purpose. Developing your sensitivity to energies in this way will help you gain judgment of what is right for you.

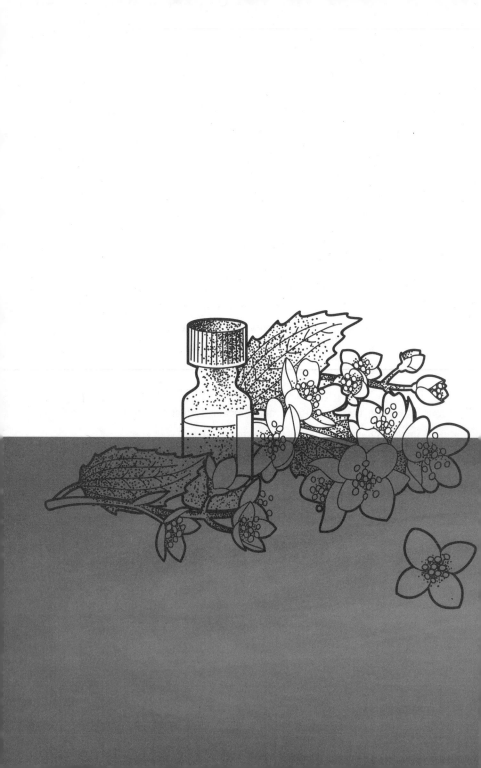

Yarrow Flower Essence

9

"I bring a collaboration of heart and mind, to fill my personal space with serenity and light, and to keep all energies in balance and at peace."

When I came across yarrow as an essence, I was instantly transported to sensations of complete serenity and calm. I had a strong sense of wellness and well-being just being in the presence of this plant. A yarrow has a strong robust stem with a head of many tiny flower clusters. I use a white plant for the essence, but yarrow can be found in a spectrum of creams, yellows, and pinks. The white color of the flowers is a symbol of simplicity, peace, security, and purity, and as such can bring that energy and those sensations in through into the essence. The yarrow flower essence is useful for times when you need to balance your energies, for new starts and new beginnings.

The way the plant expresses itself shows through its flower structure. It has a wide flower surface that looks flat but which is actually full of tiny flower clusters, and to my mind, this represents support, community, and boundaries. The fact that none of the individual flowers overpowers any of the other flowers suggests notions of fairness, equality, and wholeness. So this is a really good essence if you want help coping with pressure or if you feel that you are missing something that you just cannot put your finger on. It helps you to maintain your energetic boundaries by making you aware of your subtle bodies and bringing a sense of calm into the area around you. This is perfect for those who are highly sensitive to the atmospheres and energies that surround them.

Yarrow is a perennial and flowers throughout the summer months and dies back or becomes dormant in the autumn or winter. This gives an energetic signature that allows time for reflection and acceptance of the need to face changes and transitions.

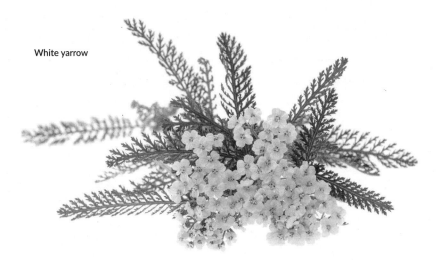
White yarrow

It gives us the opportunity to refresh and restart, and it can be particularly helpful for emotions associated with grief, loss, and of being overwhelmed, as it us aids in holding on to the idea of comfort and hope.

Other attributes given to the tiny flowers are associated with its size. If you feel isolated even when in a crowd, or if you feel empty, negative, or that you don't fit in, this essence can really support you. It allows you to clear your mind, refresh your thought patterns, and shift moods of depression and negativity and also lift brain fog. It keeps everything simple and light, rested and organized.

This plant can grow quite tall, sometimes up to around four feet in height, either in the wild or as a cultivated herb. In my experience you will often find it growing wild in hedgerows or fields. It has fern-like spiral and feathery shaped leaves which are fairly soft to touch, yet the stem is strong, and it easily props up its community of flowers. So yarrow brings the energy signature of empowering your emotions, in a soft and gentle way, and it enables you to stand tall and be strong no matter what life brings from your conditioning, environment, and current situation.

Yarrow essence allows you to come from a place of innocence and to promote harmony. If needed, it can protect your emotions by bringing emotional balance to heightened or confused energies, especially at times when you feel isolated, alone, fearful, or under attack.

Yarrow essence is perfect for a highly sensitive person (someone who is very influenced by others or by their environment). Because of the traits shared above, people who are highly sensitive will often isolate themselves from others to protect themselves emotionally or spiritually. Yarrow can also be very helpful to someone whose energies demand attention, possibly someone who comes across as having an overwhelming sense of self-worth or a lack of consideration for others.

Yarrow essence is all about balance. The white yarrow incorporates all the colors within the color spectrum, allowing you to be neutral and at ease with yourself. It allows you to be not judgmental or critical. If you find it hard to separate your thoughts and feelings, it can help you to make sense of things, to understand, to be clear, and to see a way forward. It allows you to project an aura of serenity both inwardly to yourself and outwardly to others.

This particular essence was made in group work at a private ceremony at Stonehenge in 2013, when we were celebrating World Peace Day. When you consider that an essence is the energy signature of a plant, which has been captured in the memory of water and preserved in brandy, you might see that the place, time, and circumstances in which the essence has been made can also have an impact. It can enhance the essence almost as much as the presence of the plant itself. So when making up any essence I do so in a way that will enhance the flower's inherent energy signatures.

When discussing essences with a client, I always encourage the client to think deeply about his or her needs, and to focus on what they want their essence to achieve. With this in mind, my bottles are named or given an intention that is marked on the label. Many people have described the effects of essences as magic because they can't understand or put into words the specific way in which their essence has worked for them. But this in no way belittles or removes the capability the essence brings. The client experiences a positive influence or a change for the better, and this has simply been gently accepted into the client's life, sometimes without realization.

Take a moment to think about a bottle of "magic" that you might like to have for yourself. Consider what you want your essence to achieve, but don't think in practical terms, such as wanting love, luck, or money. Bear in mind that essences work on subtle energies and inner needs. When you grasp this, it will help you focus on the essence or essences you require. By focusing on your *real* needs, you give yourself a clear direction, intention, focus, and clarity of mind—and this will help you make the right choice. You don't need to use the entire bottle in one go, so once you have used your essence, you can put it aside and use it again when you feel the need.

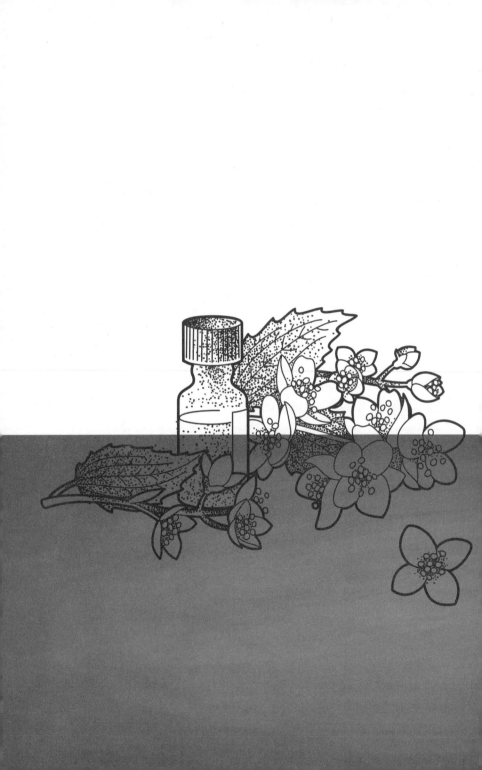

Purple Tulip Essence

10

"I welcome unconditional love, transformation,
and trust in my soul's purpose."

This essence is all about encouraging self-worth, so that we can be the best that we can be at all times. It is particularly useful when we feel insignificant or when we know that our feelings are being negated and our needs aren't being met. We may ignore our own needs at such times and consider ourselves to be unimportant when weighed against those who are around us.

When I talk about self-worth in this chapter, I am referring to the way that you feel about yourself: what *you* as an individual believe and feel, truly within yourself. If you have not done so before, you might like to challenge your perception of your own self-worth by asking yourself this: "Do I judge my self-worth against others, or can I honestly just be myself?"

Purple tulip essence is about being an individual who is confident and capable of recognizing and understanding your own inward needs and acting on them accordingly. Looking at the way that a tulip is formed offers an insight to its energy signature, and to the reason this essence brings the message that it does.

Tulips are formed from bulbs, and these are their power house that provide the vitality that is needed to sustain life as a flower, such as warmth, water, and nutrients. This bulb is its base of life, and it provides all the plant needs for growth and self-preservation. It all starts here, because without the bulb there is no tulip flower.

Thus the idea within the essence is to strengthen our own foundation. It represents what is going on inside us, and it is allied to the way we survive and grow. It relates our beliefs and our soul's purpose, and the way that we feel and connect with that. An interesting fact about the tulip is that each year the same bulb sprouts forth a new flower, an identical offspring of the first.

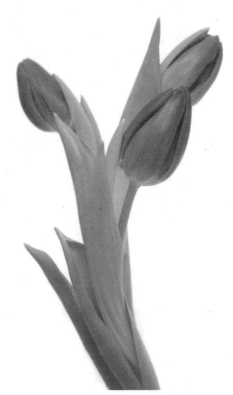

Purple tulip

Tulips come in many different colors but the one we are concentrating on here is the deep purple color. The color purple links to the crown chakra, so it suggests that we are working with the energy of that high chakra, tapping into such resources as wisdom, knowledge, spirituality, consciousness, and the subconscious.

The purple color has long been connected to royalty, importance, bravery, courage, and luxury. It is a very special color due to its rarity in nature, and that comes forward in the essence. It shows the need for us to embrace and look after our own energies and to allow ourselves to take what we need in order for us to be nurtured and supported, and to recognize that self-worth and self-esteem should not be measured against others. To me this essence allows us to feel like royalty, to feel brave, safe, and important to ourselves. It allows each of us to become a shining individual among the many other beautiful individual souls.

The tulip bulb produces a single stem with a flower. This individual flower may or may not look like the other tulips that are nearby, but it is still an individual flower. And this individual flower will grow strong and beautiful when supported from within. This is brought forward into the essence, because it allows us to feel, it allows us to connect to our heart, and it reduces our need to be critical, cynical, or judgmental of ourselves and others. It helps us balance the need to be too practical, or of being a perfectionist, or of being indecisive or impulsive. It allows us to grasp the idea of who and what we are, to feel that everything is as it should be, and to know that true comfort and contentment lie within.

If you look at the inside of a tulip and you will see the pattern of a pointed star, and this has many symbolic meanings, but when we turn to the energies of this essence, it is about connection. It can bring inspiration and recognition of our intuition, and it can gently guide us through to the right kind of sensitivity, empathy, and to our soul's purpose.

The outside of a tulip flower starts as a large closed bud, but it soon becomes a cup, a chalice, and even womb-like in shape. Imagine the tulip as a symbol for your heartfelt emotions, and that it holds and stores all that is needed, before it opens up and shares its goodies. This is a really powerful and transformative essence because, just like the plant itself, it aids in keeping us calm during periods of change so that we can feel content and relaxed in ourselves and within our own lives. It allows us to express ourselves and be open.

Eventually, as the season moves from spring to summer, the tulip lets go of its petals, dropping them back down to the earth and allowing time for reseeding. This too comes forward in the energy of essence, as it helps you to let go of all that might be holding you back, and to embrace all the future has to hold. It improves our perception and allows us to see the positive aspects of life.

Something you might want to try when working with this essence—or indeed any essence—would be to make a record of the way you want to feel. Ask yourself: which kind of positivity do you want to store in your bud? You can then ask which passions you might like to transform, or which you would like to manifest into your life. Follow this by listing the attitudes that you would like to see the end of, to let drop away, to let go of.

This is a good way of focusing your energies while working with the tulip essence, as it works in the same way as the life cycle of the flower. You can do this as often as you feel the need and whenever it feels right for you. When using the essence, you might wish to keep a journal or record of the outcomes, to enable you to judge how far you have moved with the support of flower essences. Reflection and understanding of your feelings can give you great strength and guidance. As a guide, a monthly practice might be a good time frame for this, although the choice of timing is up to you.

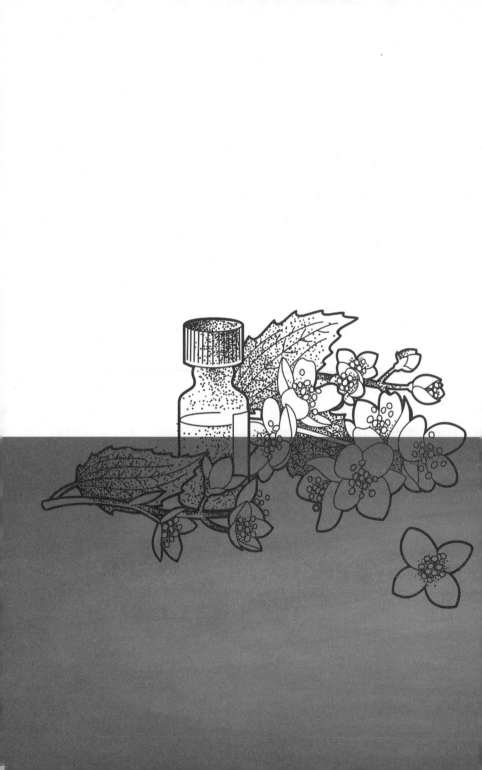

Bluebell
Flower
Essence

11

"Bluebell allows me to be rather than just do. In this quietness I find my voice and I am able to speak out from my heart."

Bluebell is an essence that everyone I meet is drawn to at some time or another. The iconic image of the bluebell itself brings feelings of being at one with the beauty and magic of Mother Nature. This certainly comes through in her flower essence.

Bluebells start to appear in the northern hemisphere in the early spring, and patches of them can hang around for many months. Sometimes we see them in vast swathes that make the earth appear to glow with their blue beauty. Usually found in woodlands or hedgerows, they make a wonderful show, and if you can visit a bluebell woodland when they are in full bloom I would encourage it.

The bluebell itself is a tall single stem with long linear leaves that droop down. The flowers are violet blue, although they can also be found in pink and white versions. The flowers come in clusters of maybe up to twenty, and they are bell shaped as their name suggests. The bells have little upturns at the bottom, making their edges look frilly. The bells face downward and move about in the breeze.

When made into an essence, these beautiful blue plants produce a mood of calmness, reassurance, stability, order, peace, and tranquility. The color and shape of the bluebell offers a good indication of the way in which this essence may strengthen us. The bell shaped flowers are open and free, facing down, which allows their energies to flow where needed. When made into an essence, this becomes particularly helpful when clarity, communication, and creativity of expression need to flow naturally. This essence allows us to feel refreshed and balanced, and it is especially important at times when you need to improve your perceptions and intuition. The essence helps to even out a roller coaster

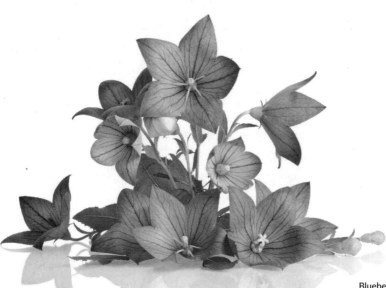

Bluebell

of emotional extremes to ensure that your inner balance is maintained at a sustainable level. Thus, this essence is ideal for those times when you are overwhelmed by anger, excitement, or when you are being taken over by great happiness or sadness.

The plant is rarely found in isolation, since its natural habitat is within a large community. Therefore, this essence helps to ease feelings of isolation or introversion. It can be useful when we lack trust or when we fear deception, or of being lost in a crowd, or when we feel the need for protection.

It is said a bluebell wood it is a sign of an ancient woodland, and this rings true of the energies and vibrational imprint of the essence, as it can reconnect us to our own unique selves. To my mind, the bluebell essence encourages us to understand our own inner world and our own subtle energies from an original, pure prospective. Think of the bluebell as our original blueprint; before it became buried over time under new plans and extensions. This is not to say there is anything wrong with change and development, but bluebell essence allows us to remember that our core foundations are still there and that they are strong. Bluebell brings a sense of unity and strength, so is perfect for those times when you feel crowded, overwhelmed, in need of stability, and when you need to be grounded and supported. If you feel that you are just keeping your head down and battling through life, bluebell will let you know you are safe and cared for.

This flower is associated with our throat chakra energies, so it enables us to communicate in a way that's appropriate and comfortable for us as an individual among many. It allows us to enjoy solitude within the company of others and to be independent and to live without being subservient. Bluebell will assist you in speaking up for yourself, especially if you feel judged by others. It does this by strengthening your confidence and self-esteem, and it helps you to learn how to look inward for guidance and strength.

Bluebell will help you release past mental or emotional patterns to bring openness and joy where previously there was darkness or fear. It aids in changing attitudes that relate to feeling low or unworthy, and it encourages self-love and self-respect.

Bluebells are mentioned in many ancient tales and they are said to grow in places where there is a deep understanding of nature. It is said they grow in places where fairies make their spells, after which they post them, along with good wishes, deep inside the flowers. It is said that if you go among the bluebells you will fall into a deep sleep, and maybe never reawaken. Leaving the myths aside, it's clear that the essence of the bluebell plant helps to rest the mind and clear away unwanted or overactive thoughts. It is an aid to meditation and relaxation, thus allowing us the emotional freedom to be in the moment. Bluebell essence will give you time to untangle and recognize your thoughts and feelings.

Use bluebell essence in a safe, undisturbed, comfortable spot in which you can rest and do this mini meditation:

Close your eyes and imagine yourself in a bluebell woodland. You are resting deep among the flowers, alone but safe.

Take a moment to witness and really see the colors of the fresh green stems and beautiful blue flowers, smell how their fragrance clears and rests your senses.

Watch as they bob, sway, and gently dance in the breeze and feel this within yourself.

Feel the calm, restful, peaceful colors engulf you, and feel your body connected with and supported by the earth.

Feel your burdens drop away, and feel your mind clear as if a bell is ringing, clearing away mind chatter or noise.

Rest, breathe deeply, and know your dreams and hopes are safe and that they are being nurtured deep within.

Feel an ancient wisdom connect and support you, and feel the love and encouragement around you.

Rest and just be in the moment, totally relaxed, calm, and content.

Breathe in the area you are visualizing and feel that you are there and try to remain for as long as feels comfortable.

Then when rested and ready start to move your physical body, gently open your eyes.

Now how do you feel?

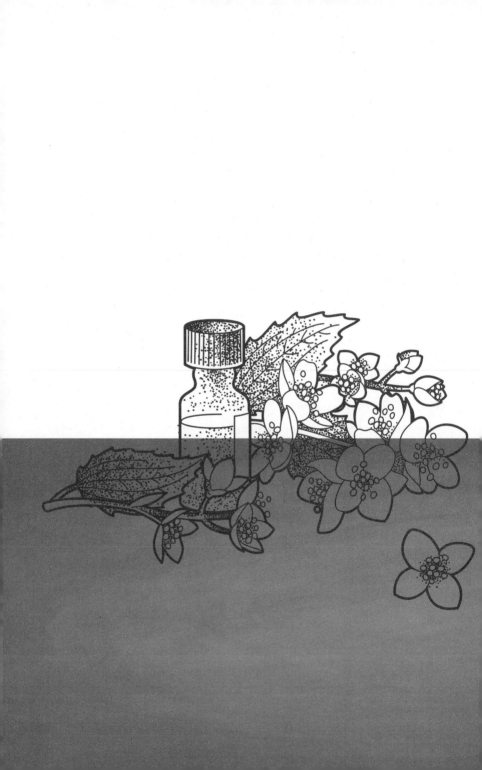

Camellia
Essence

12

"I am all that I can be, all I need to be, and all I should be. My path unfolds out into the world and brings possibilities, experiences, and positive attitudes."

To me this essence embodies all the positive qualities that we seek, because this essence can nurture our heart center and reconnect us to the heart of our being. Camellia allows our ideas to emanate from our hearts when we need to make decisions by aiding us to find common sense and calmness. She soothes our energies and brings great comfort while we are on our path through everyday life.

A camellia has many varieties and colors. It is a strong shrub with beautiful evergreen leaves. It has a strong root system that enables it to survive and to go on producing flowers and heavy dense foliage year after year. To me this comes forward in the essence, because camellia essence allows balance to be brought, allowing you to see and understand your true potential. It calms indecisiveness, improves your ability to draw on patience when you need it, and it creates serenity. So this essence is perfect for times where you feel unsettled, frustrated, confused, or energetically wired.

The plant that I have used to create all my camellia essences was very young when I first came across it, and yet it already had huge cup-shaped buds that opened to produce the most amazingly colored display of flowers. The buds started as a deep red and lightened in color as time went on, transforming into a warm orange with a bright yellow center, then finally through a lighter red to orange and brown, before closing up while drying and disappearing back to the earth. For me the beauty of the huge buds and their transformation comes forward in the essence.

The character of this essence is that it brings confidence to decision making, enhances creativity, and gives women who use it a sense of their own femininity. It raises intuition, prevents

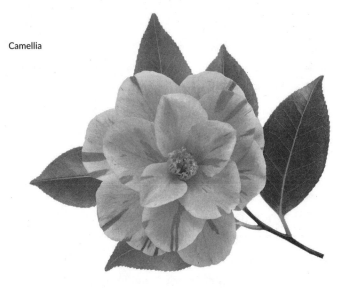

Camellia

negative thinking, and allows us to rid ourselves of unwelcome habits. It allows us to accept or reject whatever possibility opens up to us, with questioning our confidence or ability to pick the right thing. When the bloom finally opens, it may drop and dry up quickly or it may hold on to its beauty for weeks. Sometimes the flowers will fight through the early frosts, sometimes they can tolerate a little too much sun—but each bloom lasts as long as it is meant to. Thus the life cycle of the flower varies according to the circumstances that it finds itself in.

This comes forward in the essence, as each flower and its cycle has its own timing, which reminds us that as we go through life, everything happens at the right time. It isn't worth living in the past or the future, so this essence allows us to live in the present moment. It allows us to unlink from looking backward and forward in hurtful ways; it allows us to link closely to circumstances surrounding relationships with others. This essence suggests a need to seek joy, happiness, self-belief, satisfaction, and contentment.

Through its evergreen leaves and it ability to reproduce and grow quickly, camellia reminds us of our own ability to make things happen, but also of our tendency to dwell too deeply on some things. It can reconnect us with our sexuality and self-worth. It allows us to let go and expand our nature in perfect alignment to our feelings, keeping us supported and balanced.

Here is a visualization exercise to bring you closer to this essence.

Take a moment to "see" your body as the camellia plant. Close your eyes and imagine you are the plant.

Feel your toes, feet, and ankles as the strong roots that are deep in the soil—twisted, tangled, and complicated but strong, sturdy, and supportive of the rest of your body that stands above.

Now visualize the rest of your body, taking your time as you work upward.

See your legs as the stems of a woody and robust plant that is full of life force, enriching you with enthusiasm, vitality, passion, production, and positive possibilities for the future.

Now "watch" as the core your body becomes the branches and evergreen glossy leaves.

Expand to your vision to your arms and fingers, and keep this growing feeling around you as the height and density of the plant expands past your chest, your heart, and up and beyond your head.

In a spiritual sense, you have become the plant!

Now take a moment to rest and just be camellia. Take in all that is around to nourish you: the water, the wind, and the sun. Feel your feet planted firmly on the earth.

You then need to feel buds pop up and expand all over you. Acknowledge where they are on your body. These may be associated to a part of your physical body that you are happy with or some part of your body that is sick or out of sorts.

Alternatively, these buds may be just dotted around by your subconscious. Remember that you are working with the ethereal rather than the physical, so take some time to label these buds, to name them as emotions. Keep it simple to start with: happy, sad, angry, frustrated, joyful, playful, mischievous, nervous, unsettled, fearful, peaceful, determined, enthusiastic or excited.

Once each of your buds has a name, allow them to open into flowers. Now you need to decide whether you will hold them within your core or let them drop to the ground, ready for transformation or decay. If you are holding onto painful or negative passions, you may need to drop them, just as a plant loses the things it finds heavy, diseased, or no longer needed.

When you have named all your visualized blooms, make a list of them, noting those you want to keep in bloom and those you would prefer to let drop to the earth and be transformed. In this way, you copy what the camellia does by allowing the positive traits to increase and the negative ones to drop away. Or you can simply recognize that you have taken some time to be in the present moment, that you have been mindful of your feelings without judgment, stress, or pressure, which is a useful exercise in itself. Every time you practice naming your buds, you will obtain your own insight as to how you connect with your inner world.

As time goes by, you will learn more about essences and the way they care for us. I find this practice easy to do with the camellia plant due its structure and shape, but you can use any plant or tree that comes into your mind, as it will still help you to give buds names and characteristics.

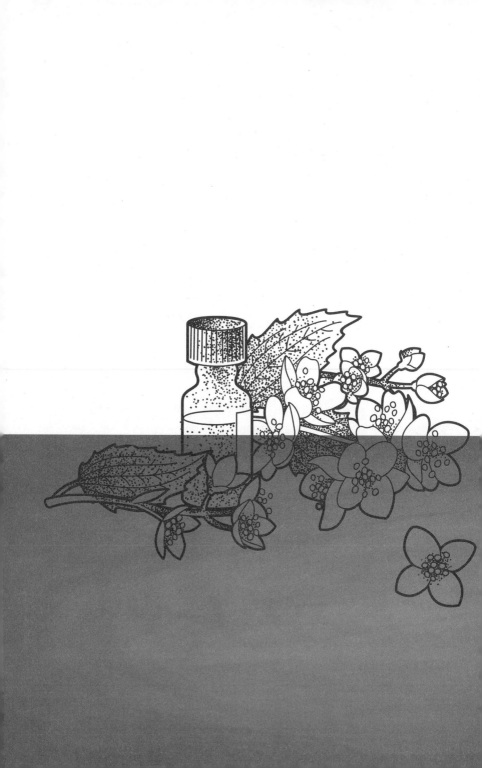

Gorse Essence

13

"I have faith that the darkness will lift and the joy and light will illuminate me."

Gorse is a really tough and resilient plant that can regrow after even the most difficult beating from bad weather or a harsh environment, and it flowers through most of the year in the northern hemisphere. It has a shrubby structure that can grow tall and wide and it is a hardy evergreen that has thorny, spiky leaves.

Gorse is common in hedgerows, the edges of parks, and cultivated lands, but you can see it all its natural splendor in heaths and moors. I made this particular essence in the place where I found the plant, when I took a break while hiking on the moors. The plant had created a shelter from the wind that is so common and ever-present on the exposed and rocky moor. So I was able to see and feel the sun through the gorse's leaves while making the essence, and of course, I was surrounded by the gorse plant itself while I was working on it.

Gorse is a useful essence when you need to combat hopelessness and when you just can't see your life getting any better, and when you are certain that you will never feel any better than you do at that moment.

Dr. Bach, who pioneered the use of flower essences, said this about gorse in 1934: "Gorse lost all hope and said, 'I can go no further: you go along, but I shall stay here as I am until death relieves my sufferings.'"

Gorse is an essence that you can turn to when you feel hopeless or for times when you can't see a light at the end of the tunnel. It is for those times when you have lost faith or when you are uncertain of life. By using the essence of gorse, you are bringing positivity to bear upon those feelings. Gorse will aid you

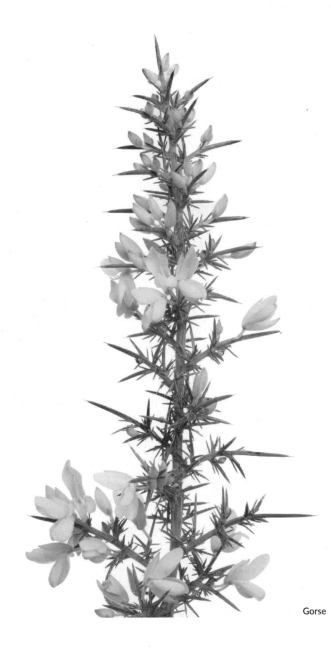

Gorse

in releasing self-doubt, it will prevent you from focusing on the negative, and it will help you focus on your way forward.

When I look at the plant and see what message there is within it to give, I can see that it is the flower that brings us its message rather than the bush itself. The flowers are usually an elongated bean shape, which reminds me of little torch lights. Is this nature's way of pointing us in the right direction? I believe so. Gorse allows us to shine light into dark times in our emotional and spiritual lives. It is an essence that will help us to change our attitudes and habits from a pessimistic state into an optimistic one.

In my experience, it works well with our solar plexus chakra and energy center, for it brings positivity and the balanced elements of confidence, capability, willpower, enthusiasm, and joy. Gorse helps us to revitalize our zest for life by finding self-esteem, drive, and determination.

Gorse essence is the essence that helps bring perfect balance to all your emotions, and it helps you to relinquish depression while it banishes a lack of faith or hopelessness. It revitalizes your ability to trust in your intuition and instinct and it gives you back your drive. Some parts of the world see gorse as a weed, and like all weeds, it grows back quickly and spreads rapidly, therefore, the essence of gorse keeps alive the determination to strive and make positive changes, even in the most uncertain and difficult circumstances.

I have found gorse essence to be particularly relevant to someone who is looking for help but who has given up looking for it. These people find themselves going through the motions of accepting new or different methods, but can't really believe in a future that embraces any change for the better. I came to include this essence in my range of therapies because so many times when asked to help I have heard words such as: "I've tried everything. You are my last hope! I have nothing to lose, do I?"

It is just such clients who are helped the most by gorse essence.

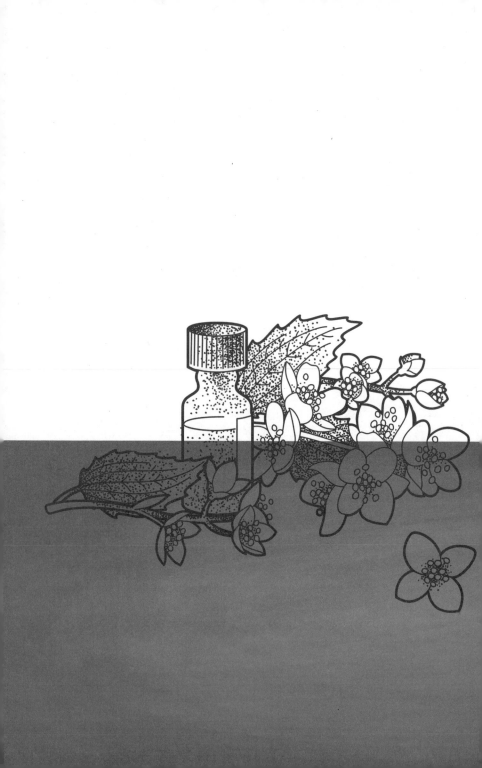

Foxglove
Essence

14

"I can create what I wish, reality is energy, and energy is the source to which I have an infinite and divine soul connection."

This plant grows in abundance in woodlands and the moors in the area where I live, and it's impossible to miss this vibrant pink plant reaching up from the forest floor. Foxglove can grow up to six feet tall and they are often weighed down with slightly bell-shaped flowers. They are known in folklore as "folks' gloves" because it's easy to put your finger inside each bell, as though each is the finger of a glove. Foxglove is also said to be connected to fairies, and it's quite easy to believe that fairies come out when there's nobody around when you see these slightly magical flowers bobbing about in the woods.

The energy and essence drawn from this plant is right for someone who wishes to make a deep connection, and who longs for contentment and peace. Its energetic aim is to provide us emotional backbone and help us recognize and realize our heart's desire from a soul level.

Foxglove self-seeds by producing millions of seeds from each plant, so this plant is often found in abundance. There is nothing understated about the energy of foxglove, as it stands tall and proud, confident in its space and purpose. This comes forward in its essence, which is great for releasing fear and anxiety, and it helps with emotions that sweep over us at times of transition and change. It encourages confidence and awareness, and it assists in bringing an openness to our perception, inner wisdom, potential, and abilities.

Note: The plant should not be ingested; it is actually poisonous since its leaves are a source of digitalis. Animals know this, so they tend to leave the plant alone but it attracts insects and bees, which help it reproduce. These insects and bees grow and prosper, and they go on to support the surrounding ecosystem.

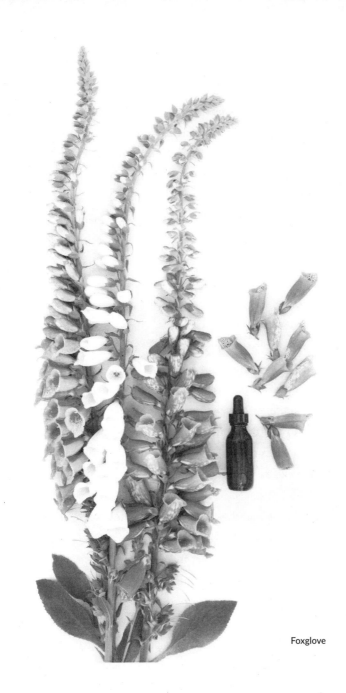

Foxglove

I'm often asked how I can make an essence that is safe to take when it has originated from poisonous plant, so this is the perfect time for me to remind you that **essences have no biological matter** inside them. When making an essence you are working with the plant's *energy*, its *life force*, and its *vibration*. In the case of the foxglove, it is important for me to choose the right plant and to do so in the right place. I don't cut these plants, so this essence is made by what's known as the indirect method (see page 24). The area where I make this essence is a natural site, protected by local authorities as a nature preserve, which limits the way that people can influence or spoil the area. The indirect method, and the protected environment of the plant, really help to maintain the power of the essence.

Foxglove essence can be used to help reconnect the soul with nature and it helps us to understand all that Mother Earth has to offer. It works with our energy centers and subtle bodies to promote an intense connection to both our physical place on earth and our higher selves within the universe. It bestows an awareness of everything around us, while allowing us to remain grounded. This essence really helps during meditation, astral travel, channeling, trance work, and exploring past lives.

When the foxglove flowers are in full bloom, they are a hive of activity and their height and color make them stand out. They so completely represent the atmosphere of summer, invoking a sense of love, joy, and happiness.

The essence helps us to overcome self-doubt and indecisiveness. It can release us from past hurts or past mistakes and it aids us in changing patterns or breaking damaging habits. It balances and realigns the heart and soul chakras, allowing us to feel the energies of unconditional and universal love. Foxglove essence brings so many qualities that we so badly need to ensure our emotional health and well-being. It brings connection to who we are, it protects us from any harmful atmospheres and energies that may be in our surroundings, and it pulls serenity, deep love, support, and positivity around us.

The foxglove message is: "I can create what I wish." This affirmation brings with it an element of trust in the future and in a positive outcome. It is a bit like the power of positive thinking, in that if we really feel we cannot achieve something, it will be very hard for us to make it work. Whereas, if we feel deep inside ourselves that we *can* succeed, even though it will take time and effort, we will get there in the end.

Some people say essences have just a placebo effect and science is unable to prove beyond reasonable doubt that they work, and yet hundreds of people report symptoms and emotional conditions improving when they use essences. If you can start to work with your whole health, trusting and knowing that there is more than can be seen with the human eye, then we are truly invoking the bounty that foxglove can bring us. It is really important to remember that essences are *not* a substitute for medical care and treatments, but a complementary tool for us to call on when we need help on physical, mental, emotional, and spiritual levels. Essences are a natural way of helping us to become all that we can be or all that we want to be.

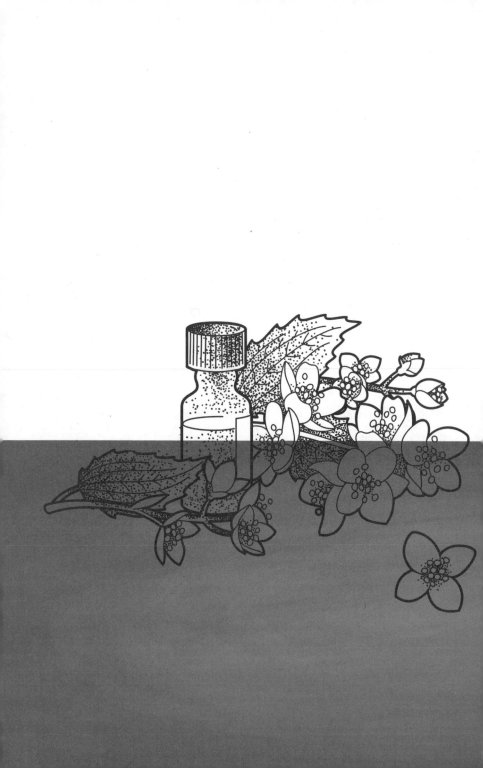

Buttercup Flower Essence

15

"I bring joy and hope. I allow my inner child to be free as I shine my light out into the world and realign my own inner resources."

The buttercup is a common flower from April through September in the United States and Britain. Many of us associate it with a game played as children, when we would pick a buttercup and shine it under a friend's chin, whereupon the light reflected from its waxy petals would tell us if that person liked butter by the strength of the color. When considering the essence, butter doesn't come into it, but it does give a clue to its vibration and life force.

Buttercup essence is an essence that allows you to shine light on a situation that encompasses negativity, loss of faith, a weakening of will power, and a lack of energy and strength. Buttercup essence can produce a constructive state of mind. It allows us to recognize that there is hope, and that the light shining is the positivity of change, giving us back any personal power that we may have lost. This essence is perfect for someone who is down, depressed, pessimistic, or who has been through a difficult situation that is holding them back or who is having difficulty in trusting that things can get better.

It is a perfect essence for allowing someone the emotional space and freedom needed to shine their unique light in the world. The energy and life force it brings is one of confidence and capability. It is a great essence for anyone who feels they are lacking confidence or who can't believe in themselves. It is great for those who fear failure, or who get anxious or distressed at the thought of trying. It combats destructive perfectionism and it combats the negative sentiments that are attached to disbelief or hopelessness.

The cup shape of the flower signifies the ability to hold on to what we need, and to release what is not needed. This happens

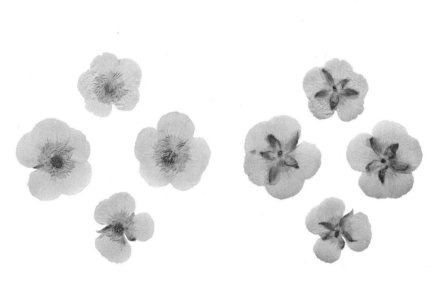

naturally when we open up to lighter emotions—just as the buttercup flower does. As it stretches its petals out, it becomes more star-like than cup-like in form, and this is a symbol of hope and a better future.

This flower represents childlike innocence and allows our energies to become more fun-loving and emotionally playful, while it is busy increasing our positivity. It allows us to see and feel things without prejudice or judgment, and just as the flower may grow abundantly throughout a meadow, it brings the energy of a supportive family or community and abundance. It can dispel fear and bring courage and self-expression. It also helps combat emotions linked to loneliness, isolation, self-worth, and lack of fulfillment.

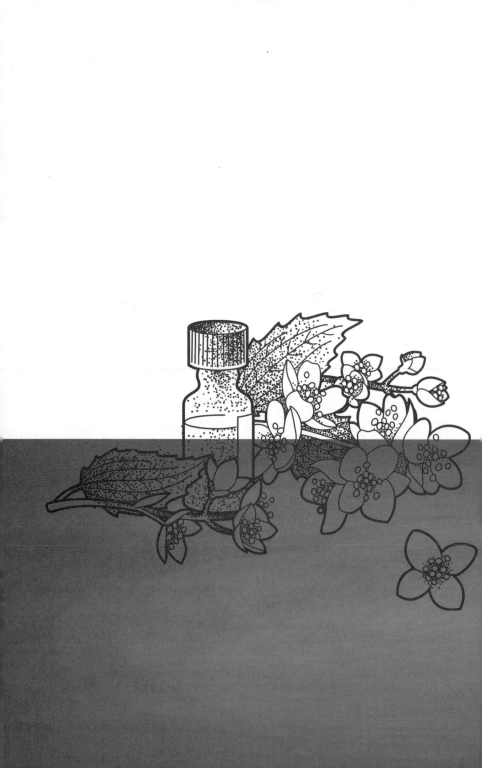

Lavender
Essence

16

"To know, to trust, to connect, to feel at one; I can feel clear, cool, calm, and safe as I relax and rejoice in my space within other spaces with no worries at all."

M any people love and connect with lavender as a plant, so it is probably not surprising to discover that the essence is very calming to our energies and emotions. Lavender is commonly used in aromatherapy oils and bath soaps for its calming effect. But the flower essence can be so much more than how it has been traditionally understood. The plant's vibrational value as an essence works on a deep level, getting to the source of what is keeping us from a calmer state of being. It works on balancing the emotions when they are intense or overwhelming. When we feel as though we are on an emotional roller coaster due to overwhelming excitement, sadness, exhilaration, or severe disappointment, lavender essence will help us come back to our center, by calming those feelings and finding a point that is naturally balanced for us.

There are a variety of lavender plants, and they vary in species and colors, but the one I used to make this essence is traditional English lavender. It has a dense shrub like lower area that has silvery leaves, and then there are long stems that produce the vibrant and fragrant purple flower heads. Although known and used in many cultures for many purposes, lavender is perfect for soothing overstretched nerves and tension. Therefore, if you feel agitated, angry, or upset it will help restore your inner peace. It brings a sense of serenity and calm by harmonizing negative emotions. Lavender brings a level of balance when your energy field is in need of a deep cleansing, or when you need to clear excessive stimulation. This makes lavender a great choice for those who quickly become overwhelmed by energies of others, and who are very empathetic or sensitive to their surroundings.

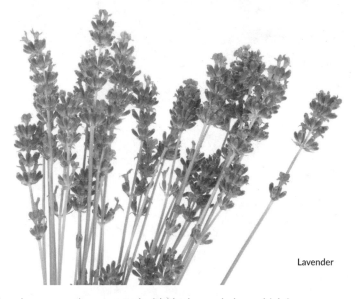

Lavender

Lavender essence is connected with the brow chakra, which is often referred to as our mind center or third eye. If this center is out of balance, a person's ability to separate reality from fantasy is usually hindered. When in balance, this chakra shows a dynamic, interesting, inspirational person, but when it is out of balance it shows an introverted, forgetful, and sometimes fearful person.

Lavender will help you reconnect to your true self, by cooling emotions, giving you mental clarity, and allowing you time to rest your energies. It is a great essence to keep you in the present moment. It is a wonderful essence to help you connect with your spiritual self or to prepare you for meditation.

Lavender connects us with our intuition, it prevents over-analysis, rigidity, and over-thinking. It allows us to be creative, imaginative, playful, and even a little dreamy. It allows an awareness of reality, and is equally helpful for people who are lost in their thoughts, and aids in balancing that space so they can function in a more practical way on a day to day basis.

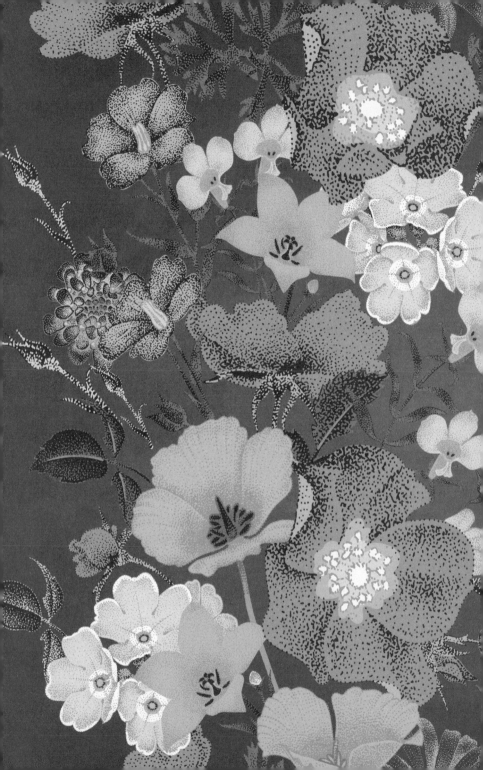

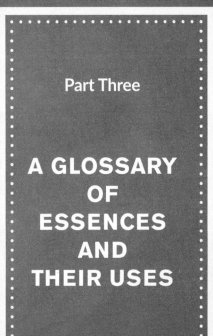

Part Three

A GLOSSARY OF ESSENCES AND THEIR USES

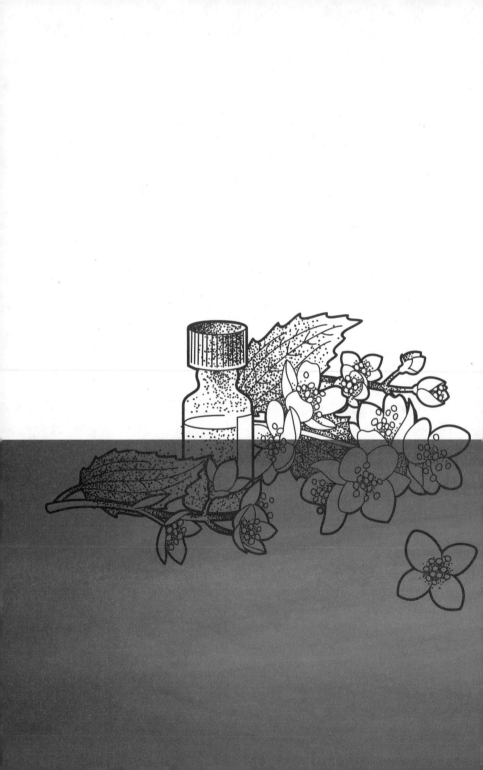

Essence
Treatment
Keywords

17

These are commonly used essences, along with some keywords to help understand their uses. The keywords indicate in some instances the problem you wish to treat; in other instances the keyword indicates a benefit from the essence. Essences, as mentioned earlier, can also be used in combination. You will certainly find more than one keyword that resonates with you.

On your journey to becoming more attuned to your personal vibration, your health, and your well-being, remember the words of Dr. Bach—the seven moods that cause disease and suffering are fear, uncertainty, loneliness, lack of interest, over-sensitivity, over-concern for others, and despair. Read these keywords with those seven basic dysfunctions in mind.

Keywords for Use

Agrimony—inner turmoil

Almond—moderation

Alpine Aster—fear of death

Alpine Lily—self-assured feminine identity

Angelica—spiritual guidance and protection

Apple—peaceful clarity and healthfulness

Aspen—fear of something unknown

Avocado—training and responsiveness

Banana—cooperation

Beech—intolerance

Black Eyed Susan—repression of trauma

Blackberry—procrastination

Borage—depression, lack of confidence

Buttercup—low self worth

Calla Lily—gender confusion

Centaury—not being able to say no

Cerato—lack of self-belief, uncertainty

Chamomile—moodiness and irritability

Cherry—healing past trauma

Cherry Plum—fear of losing control

Chestnut Bud—not learning from experience

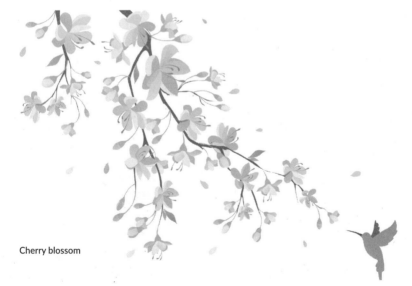

Cherry blossom

Chicory—possessive and clingy

Clematis—daydreaming, not being in the present

Coconut—transcendence

Columbine—lack of creativity, mid-life crisis

Corn—liveliness

Cosmos—disorganized communication

Crab Apple—cleansing

Dandelion—tense, over-worked, overly driven

Date—tender sweetness

Dogwood—physical awkwardness, accident prone

Echinacea—poor sense of self identity

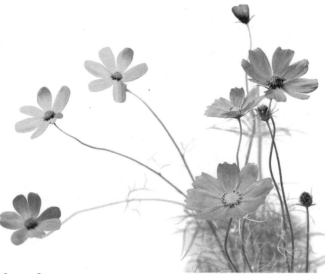

Cosmos flowers

Forget-Me-Not

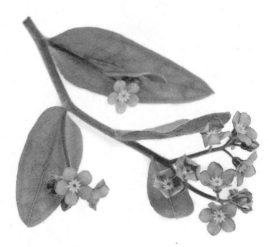

Elm—overwhelmed with responsibility

Evening Primrose—feelings of rejection

Fig—adaptability

Forget-Me-Not—karmic connections

Gentian—restores faith

Goldenrod—social awareness, peer pressure

Gorse—pessimism and hopelessness

Grape—love and wholeness

Hawthorn—type A personality, hostility

Heather—self concern

Hibiscus—sexuality

Holly—envy and jealousy

Honeysuckle—stuck in the past

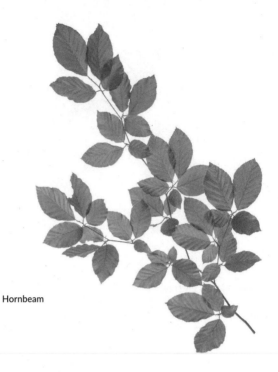

Hornbeam

Hornbeam—obsessiveness

Hyssop—body-soul integration

Impatiens—impatience

Indian Paintbrush—low vitality, exhaustion

Lady Slipper—chakra balancer

Larch—lack of confidence

Larkspur—self-aggrandizement

Lavender—nervous energy, insomnia

Lemon—mental fatigue

Lettuce—calmness

Lilac—sadness, isolation, alienation

Lotus—lack of humility

Lupine—selfishness, greed

Mallow—insecure in relationships

Mimulus—overly fearful of daily life events

Monkshood—spiritual trauma

Mugwort—hysteria, fantasy, or projection

Mustard—down and gloomy for no reason

Nasturtium—depletion of life force

Oak—for the person who works until exhaustion sets in

Olive—exhaustion

Orange—enthusiasm

Peach—nurturing

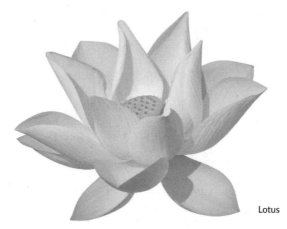

Lotus

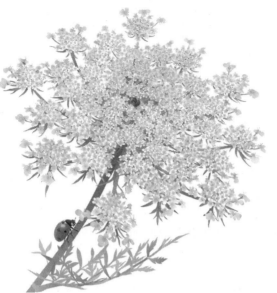

Queen Anne's Lace

Pear—peace and emergency

Peppermint—mental lethargy

Pine—guilt

Pineapple—confidence

Pink Yarrow—lack of emotional clarity

Primrose—ingratitude, joylessness

Queen Anne's Lace—spiritual insight

Raspberry—sensitivity and kindness

Red Chestnut—worry about loved ones

Rock Rose—fright

Rock Water—rigidity

Rosemary—forgetfulness

Rue—scattered or confused

Sage—inability to see purpose in life

Scleranthus—indecision

Shasta Daisy—over-intellectualization

Snapdragon—verbal aggression

Spinach—youthfulness and trust

St. John's Wort—psychic vulnerability, depression

Star of Bethlehem—shock

Strawberry—grounding and dignity

Sunflower—"dark night of the soul"

Sweet Chestnut—despair

Tansy—lethargy, procrastination

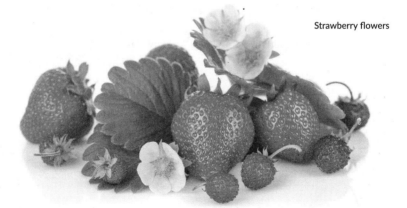

Strawberry flowers

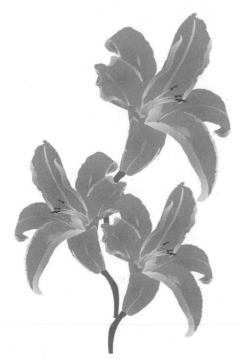

Tiger Lily

Tiger Lily—excessive yang, aggression

Tomato—fearlessness

Valerian—negative emotions, especially anger

Vervain—over-enthusiasm, fanaticism

Vine—domineering, inflexibility

Violet—profound shyness

Walnut—protection

Water Violet—grief

White Chestnut—busy mind

Wild Oat—needing a sense of direction

Wild Rose—apathy

Willow—self-pity and resentment

Yarrow—overly vulnerable

Zinnia—workaholic, lack of humor

Zinnia

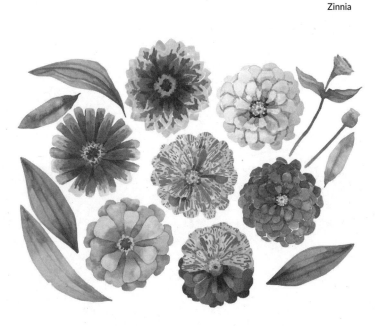

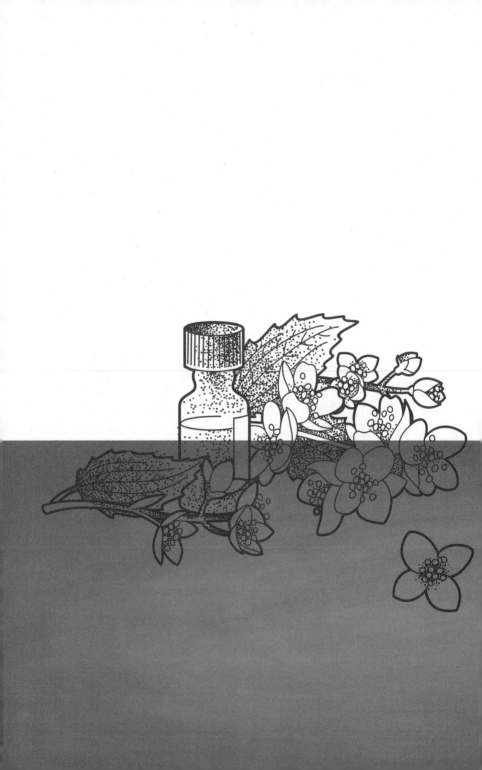

How and When to Use Essences

18

You don't need to be suffering or in a bad way before considering using an essence. Essences can be used on a daily basis to maintain healthy balance; you do not need to be in a negative state of mind to find them helpful. It is usual to call on essences in difficult situations, but they can be used to enhance and our health and well-being in many different ways. Most importantly, they can be used to keep our chakra energies in balance, for I believe that this life energy balance is what allows us to make the most of our personalities, talents, traits, habits, and behaviors.

After so much experience working on myself and with clients, I now find myself seeing the world in the vibrations, colors, and the associated meanings of flowers, plants, and trees. This means that when I meet someone during the course of my working day, I often find myself considering the flowers or plants that may help to make their lives easier. Strangely enough, even during conversation I find the person already has had a recent connection to a particular plant. It may be that someone bought them a potted plant or perhaps a new plant has appeared in their garden. It could be they visited somewhere new and were blown away by the beauty or severity of a natural habitat. So I now follow my intuition and use the knowledge I have obtained, and my desire to help reconnect people with who they are, to allow them to feel the best they can on a daily basis, and for them to get the most from life.

When I started to become attuned to the vibrations and more aware of my feelings, I began to understand how I could influence my own emotions in a gentle way by using essences. When this happened, some people thought I was living in a dream state, and that being so in touch with my intuitive and emotional self was contrary to living in the "real" world. Being in tune with your emotions is both a challenge and a gift. We are all used to seeing each other overworked, overwhelmed, very busy, and distracted by multiple daily demands. We are not used to seeing our family, friends, and coworkers in a state of peace—so it can seem a little dreamy and unrealistic. It's been all too easy for us to deny and neglect our inner needs. But when we recognize our emotional and mental state and then use essences as a natural tool, it can put us back together.

So if you are being called to by a flower, plant, or tree, it is quite simply nature's way of caring for you. There's an old saying, "Stop and smell the roses," always a metaphor for not missing out on the good things in life. But in this case, *literally stop and smell the roses!* Listen to your feelings, take appropriate guidance, and obtain information where needed and remember that we all have the ability to use our intuition. We can all keep our chakras, our subtle bodies, our energy centers, and the seat of emotions in balance. Such a sense of harmony and emotional well-being is not a state of negativity or stupidity, but a better alternative to feeling stressed, lost, upset, and out of balance.

How to Take Essences

Many producers and practitioners will give their own guidance on taking essences, written on the bottle labels, or in the information that accompanies their products, or through consultations. My advice is to begin taking essences in moderation; be kind to your energies and start by taking a few drops directly under your tongue. If you are unsure of the taste or feeling the essence gives you, add a few drops of the essence to water and drink it very slowly.

I would suggest that you take essences at the start of your day. Give your body some time to adapt to the newness, and stick with an essence for a while to give yourself time to absorb its energies. My general suggestion is four weeks. If you take an essence for a particular intention or purpose, you will definitely need time for your energy fields to take it on board, especially if you are starting from a point of serious suffering. So time is an important part of the process. If you need more time, that's fine too. For example, if I am working on a tricky job or want to achieve something in particular, I would take an essence that is designed to give me the result I need. If I needed to bring my thoughts, feelings, or energies to a heightened state, I would take more of the essence attached to bring this about. It's usually the case that the person who is taking the essence finds out for themselves when it has done its job and when it is no longer needed.

Essences can also be used as sprays or misters that you can use on your subtle bodies—such as in the bath, or in room misters. They can be added to your favorite bath or body product. I've even been known to use them in garden, on food, or in my mop and bucket when cleaning. You can use them in any way that feels right to you.

So to summarize: Use essences for upsets and distress, relationship issues, tension and strain, despondency and sadness, feelings of negativity or when coping with change and challenges.

Use them for a lack of self-confidence, fear, worry, lack of focus, lack of direction, and feelings of disempowerment.

How to Store Essences

Essences usually come in dark glass bottles or sprays and it's best to keep them air tight so they do not evaporate or take on foreign matter. Keep them out of direct sunlight and away from strong smells, and keep them away from other products and environmental influences such as electronic equipment. Essences are made from natural life forces and are themselves sources of energy, so they need to be kept safe. I would suggest that you keep them out of the reach of pets, children, and away from open flames for fear of them being broken or destroyed (and the alcohol content in them is flammable). If you want your essence to be available to you next time you need it, it's best to keep it safe.

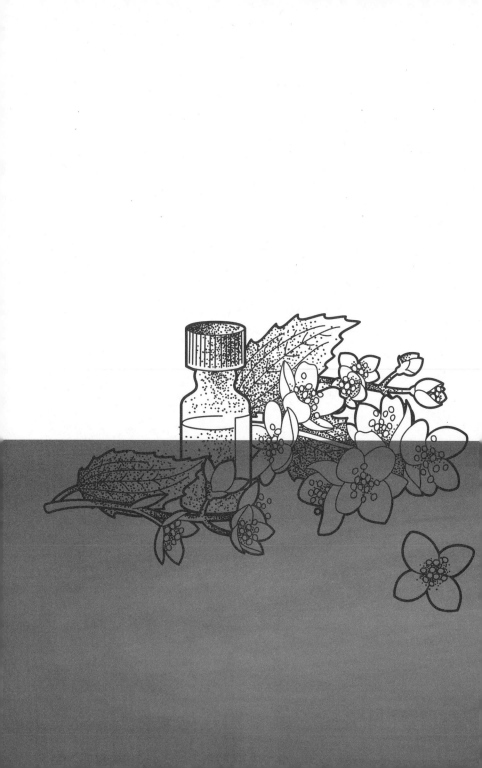

Essences
in Action:
Case Studies

19

As a holistic practitioner with a speciality in treating with flower essences, I have had the honor to help a number of clients. These two case studies are presented here to show you the power of healing with flower essences. I have changed the names of my clients to protect their identity, and they have graciously given me permission to use their stories.

Case Study One—Alison

Situation: Anxiety and Fear

Alison came to me looking for help with a variety of issues, including anxiety, fatigue, and fear of going out and being in crowds of people. This woman had been struggling with these problems for at least five years. She was being supported by her doctor, and she had consulted him before seeing me; he agreed that trying flower essences would be a positive move.

Alison had not taken essences before and she was skeptical as to how they could help, but was willing to try. I always start by talking through the client's circumstances. Alison lived on her own after her divorce, which had happened three years earlier. She had a number of physical conditions for which she was undergoing treatment, but her main complaint was fatigue. The consultation took place at her home, so she wouldn't become stressed and upset by having to go to a new place for our first meeting. She had been through a number of traumatic events over the last five years, and we discussed in detail how she felt about those, before revisiting her current status.

Task:

The number of issues that needed addressing required a combination of essences that would allow us to gently start working on each area, and then to address deeper issues as they were to arrive. I work with about 400 essences, and she was open to methods to narrow down our selection. We talked about the colors, shapes, and flowers to which she was drawn and ones she disliked; we did this using picture cards. In the end, this gave us a smaller number of essences to work with. We then went through the dowsing process to narrow the choices further, after which I used my knowledge on how each essences could work, based on the way she wanted to feel, before I created her first dosage bottle.

Action:

The dosage bottle included aspen, which is used to support someone who is afraid without knowing why. Star of Bethlehem is used for shock, and this would gently support her feelings in the transition of change. This essence helped her cope with the shock and adjustment to her new vibrations. I added buttercup essence to help her recognize that there is hope and to rebuild the energy centers that are attached to strength of emotions, so that she would begin to feel more capable and confident. Last but not least, I added red geranium, because we were working with fear and the need for security and stability in life. Red geranium is focused upon the root chakra—her foundation. She was to take a few drops every day, and more if she had a sudden surge of any of the negative feelings that she was desperate to reduce and remove.

I encourage my clients to name their bottles or give them an affirmation, and Alison named her bottle, "I am able."

Result:

The essence was taken as suggested above, and Alison kept a notebook of the results. I have reported the outcomes here in the Alison's own words.

"**Week one**—I instantly felt better using the essences you gave me. I've taken them a lot but I am finding that I'm more confident and now I can tell people what's wrong when I'm not coping.

"**Week two**—I still have all the physical pain but I'm managing it differently. My doctor said I sounded more positive and upbeat. I told him about our session.

"**Week three**—I was able to go out for coffee with a friend this week and it was so much fun. I was nervous but I know I can do this now. I'm going to practice lots.

"**Week four**—I reflected this week and had a moment where I can't remember when I last felt anxious, as the anxiety has just gone, although I can't remember exactly when this happened."

Outcome:

A really positive outcome for Alison, who is no longer a skeptic. The essences in the first and subsequent dosages have, in her words, given her the emotional strength to get her life back.

Case Study Two—Beryl

Situation: Insomnia

Beryl came to me asking for help because she was finding it hard to get a good night's sleep. When working with essences I'm not trying to "cure" the physical condition or create an outcome as such, but to improve the client's emotional state. This in turn may improve other aspects of the client's life, which allows the client to function in the here and now, to see the positive in life, and to be content. In this case the goal was to find the cause underlying her inability to sleep.

So I spent some time with Beryl in order to understand her lifestyle. She is a busy consultant working with clients six days a week. She has grown children who do not live at home, and she has a partner with whom she is in a happy relationship. She explained that she loved her job and didn't think she had anything going on at home that should stop her from sleeping. We discussed how she felt as a result of not sleeping well and the words that came up were lack of motivation, feeling sad, irritable, and an emotional heaviness in her head. She felt as though she had lots on her mind but couldn't pinpoint what exactly was bothering her. She was also concerned that being so tired would make it difficult for her to help all the people she had booked at her job, and she was worried about letting them down.

We also discussed how she felt when she was *trying* to sleep, and the description included overwhelmed, thinking of what happens if she doesn't sleep, and stressed because she feared that not sleeping would impact the next day. She felt frustrated because this had been going on day after day, for over a year. We discussed what she would like her essence to achieve and what was her "intention," because for me, intention would be the key to finding the right essence. Beryl simply said that she wanted to sleep.

I asked Beryl to consider how she thought she would feel if she could sleep well again, and she came up with feelings of happiness, a clear head, zest for life, feeling capable, strong and productive, which in turn would lead to fulfillment and contentment that she had been feeling before this problem had appeared. She found it difficult to express in words the way she felt—which is a common phenomenon when clients start to work on themselves. The logical mind starts to analyze the words that come out, which means the client either suppresses or does not acknowledge his or her true feelings, due perhaps to pride, embarrassment, or fear. It's a fact that the more a client works with essences the more he or she becomes comfortable, and thus it becomes easier to prescribe the right essence.

Task:

In this case, a flower had already come to mind while Beryl and I were talking—then to my surprise, she actually mentioned it! She said she had been trying lavender essential oil as an aid in physical relaxation because she had heard it helps sleep, but for her it had not worked. Rather than use this as the sole confirmation, I decided to confirm my thoughts by dowsing, which led to a positive reaction for lavender. We then chatted about how she had heard about lavender as a sleep aid. She confirmed she had been at a garden center when she had spotted a huge display that was covered with busy bees, and the shopkeeper had told her how good lavender is. She had then done some research online and found that products containing lavender were used for sleep.

Action:

Together we decided to try lavender essence for four weeks. Beryl drank the essence in one or two drops in water through the day, and put one or two drops directly under her tongue about an hour before she went to bed. I explained that the plant would connect and show its vibration as we had already discovered through dowsing.

Lavender essence has the ability to balance emotions and it brings a sense of inner peace. This seemed really important since Beryl had mentioned frustration, worry, and being irritable. Lavender essence allows you to be in the moment, to live life in the full, and connect with your feelings. It is a powerful essence that will allow your intuitive mind to work without getting into a battle with your logical mind. It also aids in not being self-critical or over-thinking.

Despite the fact that Beryl had told me she loved her job, she was working long hours, and her energies were mixing with those of her clients; Beryl was a "sponge" and the energies of others were becoming absorbed into her own energy centers. Lavender is protective in a cleansing way, so it could help her to be more "in the present" with her clients and separated from them when they left. To my mind, this would help her to achieve her intention.

I encourage my clients to name their bottles or give them an affirmation, and Beryl called this bottle "Calm, clear, and complete."

Result:

The essence was taken as suggested above and the results here are in Beryl's words.

"**Week one**—feeling calm and happy but still not sleeping. Noticing how I feel more, became quite aware of what's putting me off balance—the triggers. This allows me to deal with them.

"**Week two**—realized I'm not worrying about customers any more. I feel more supported and I have now managed one full night's sleep.

"**Week three**—sleeping quite well and taking everything in my stride. People are noticing I look relaxed. Still feeling calm but actually "feeling" it, don't even notice that I'm doing it now. Until you ask!

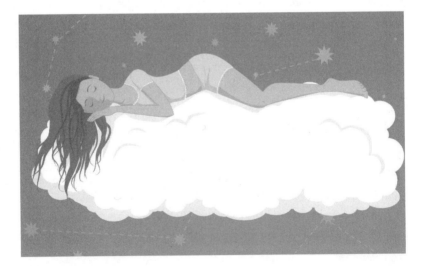

"**Week four**—sleeping every night. Have clear head. Am getting things done with ease. Am finding decision-making easier. I feel energized and happy. Still calm. Life feels so much more complete and yet the only thing I have changed is taking essence. You have helped me to reconnect."

Outcome:

I did not do anything to cure Beryl—the lavender did! Now Beryl takes lavender during busy work weeks, but she sometimes forgets (her words) to take it, which probably indicates that her need for it is lessening. She continues to use essences for many other purposes, as her essence journey continues. She feels more positive about her life and her feelings, as well as those of the people who are around her.

Hampton Roads Publishing Company

...for the evolving human spirit

Hampton Roads Publishing Company publishes books on
a variety of subjects, including spirituality, health,
and other related topics.
For a copy of our latest catalog, call (978) 465-0504 or visit our
distributor's website at *www.redwheelweiser.com*. You can also sign up
for our newsletter and special offers by going to
www.redwheelweiser.com/newsletter